Asthma - Biological Evidences

Edited by Celso Pereira

Published in London, United Kingdom

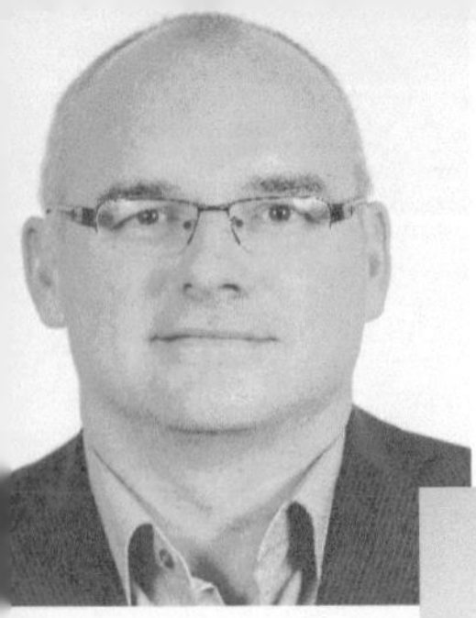
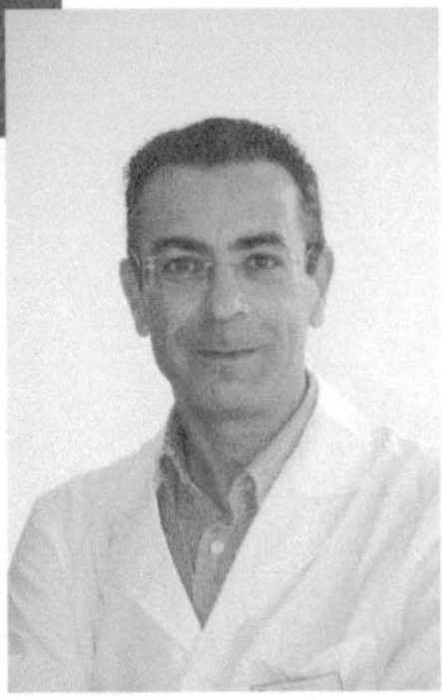
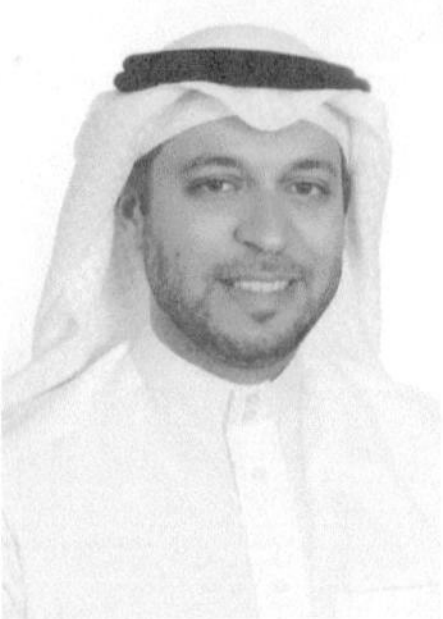
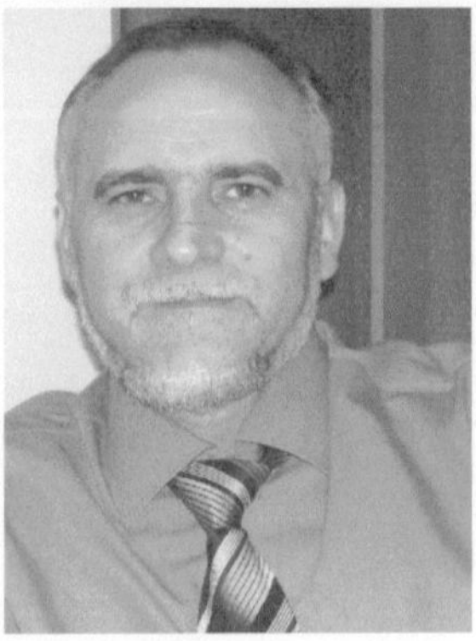
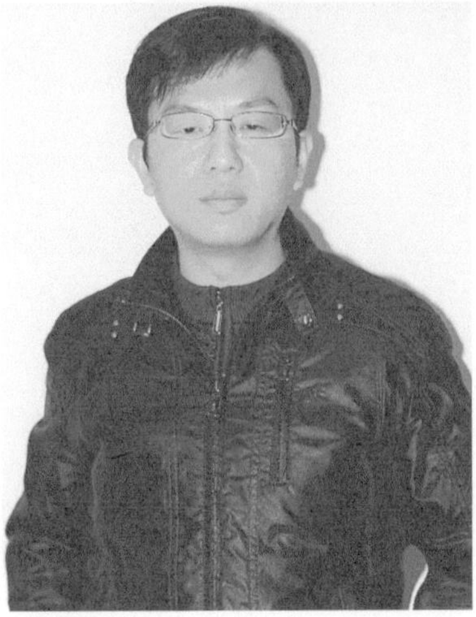
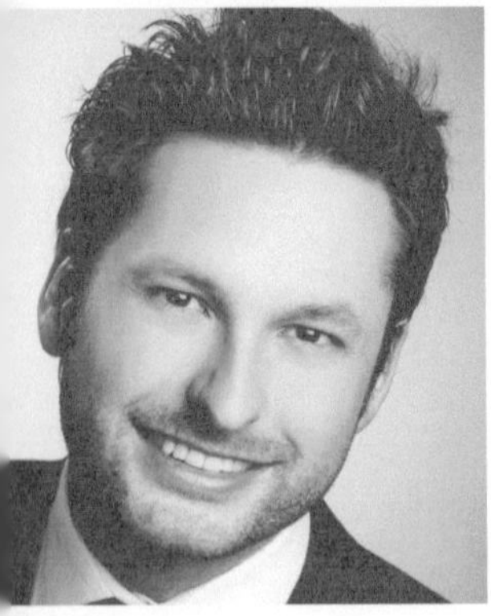
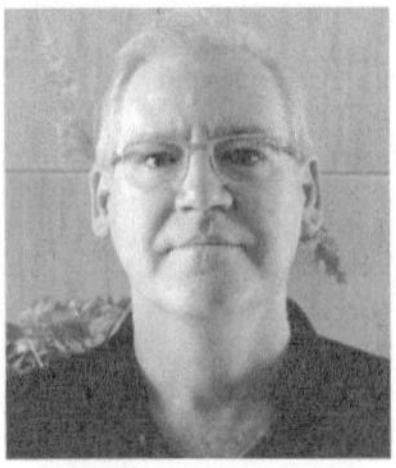

IntechOpen

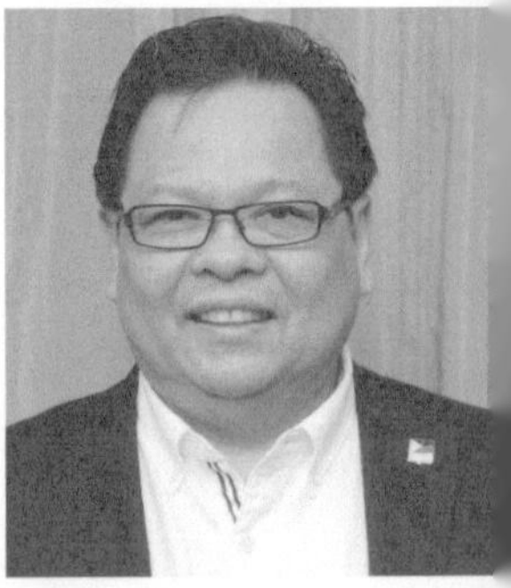
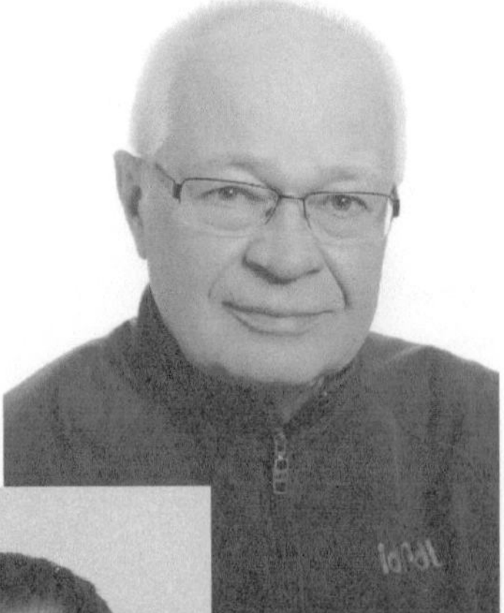
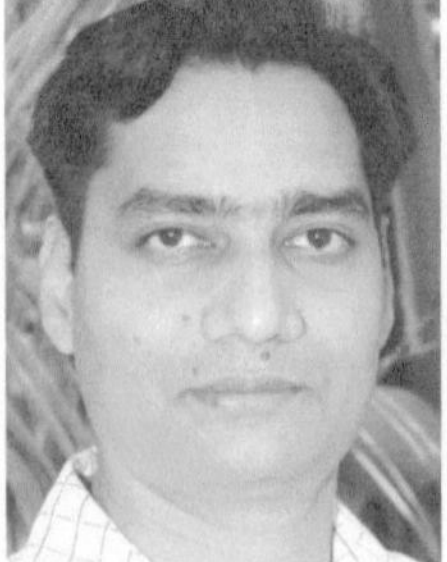
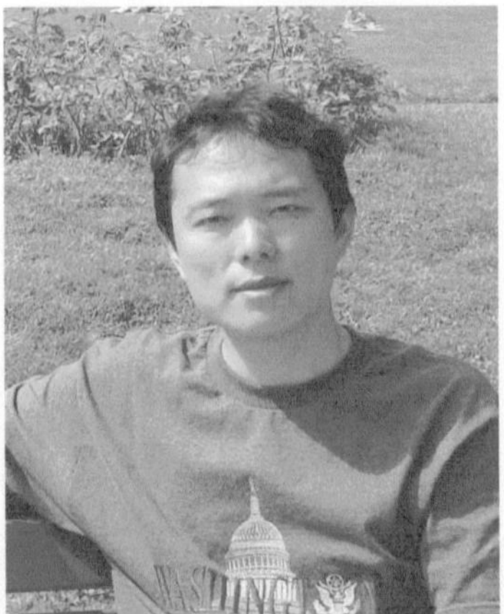
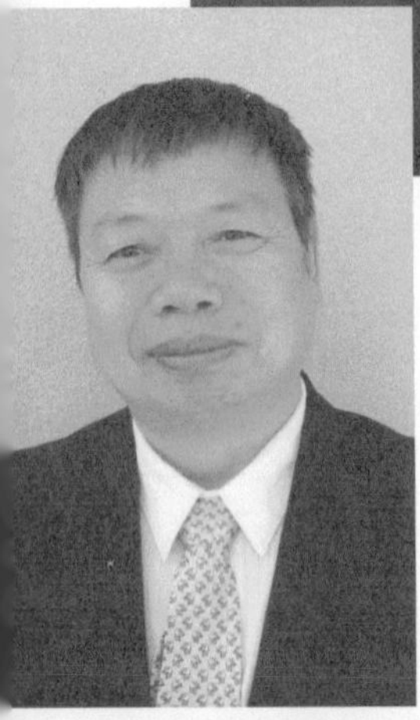
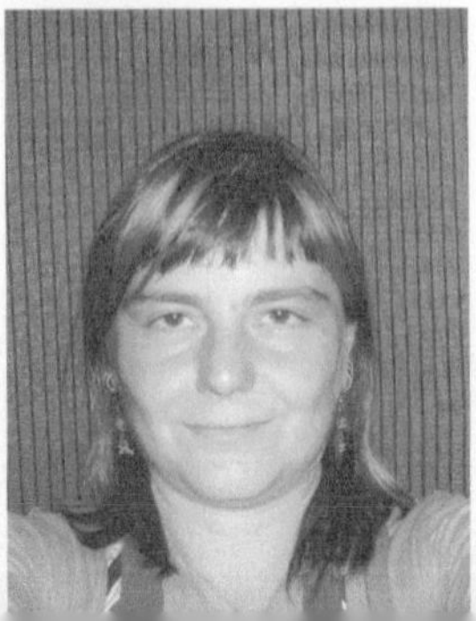

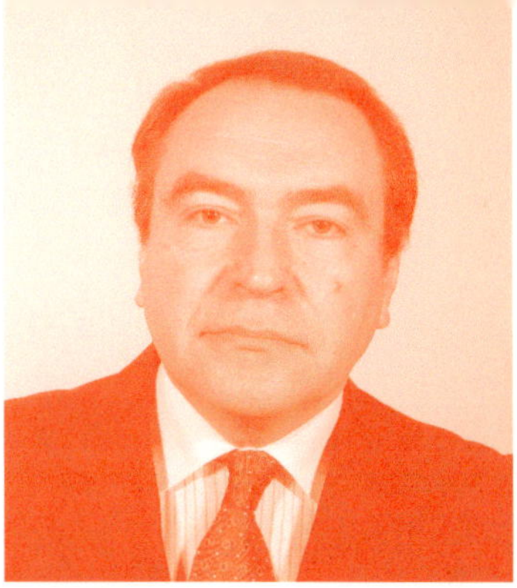

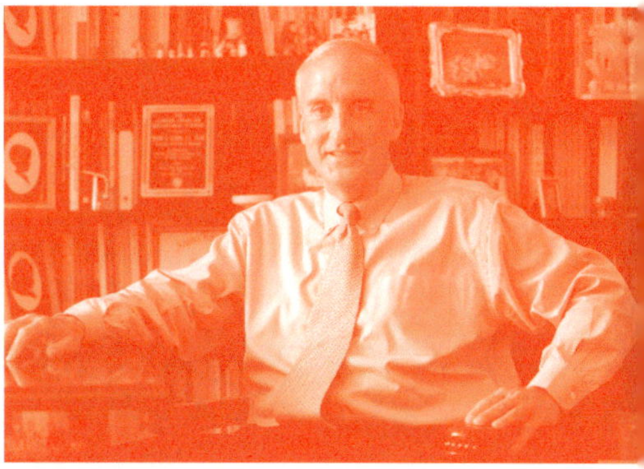

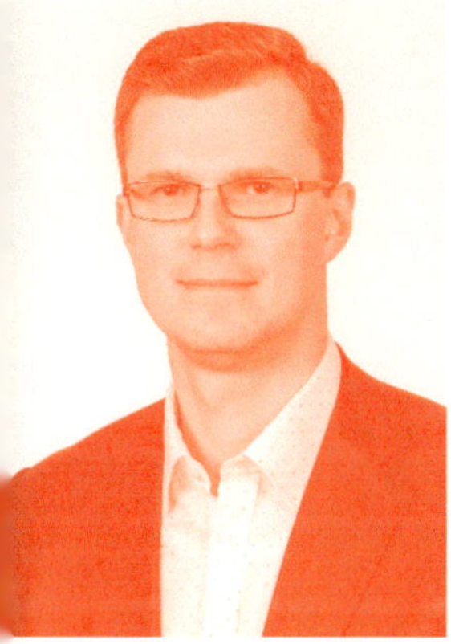

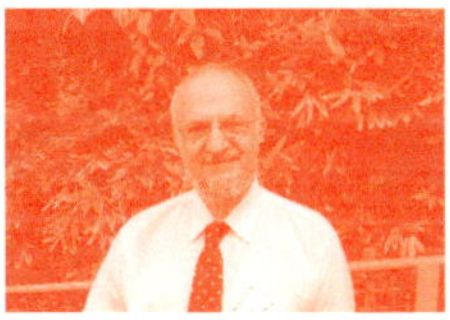

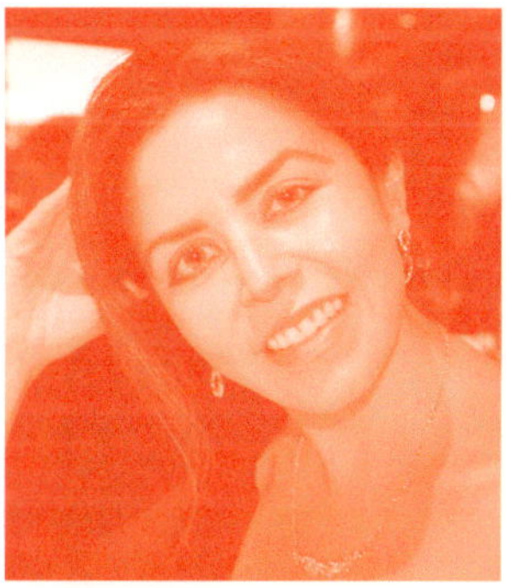

Supporting open minds since 2005

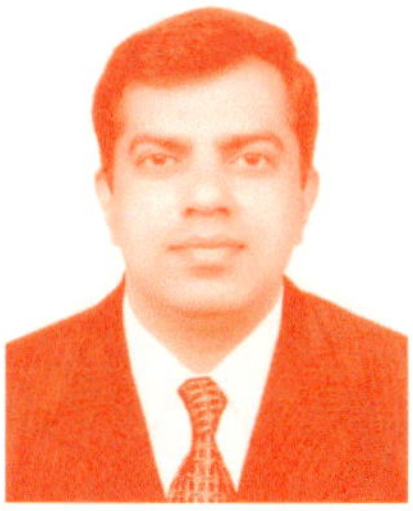

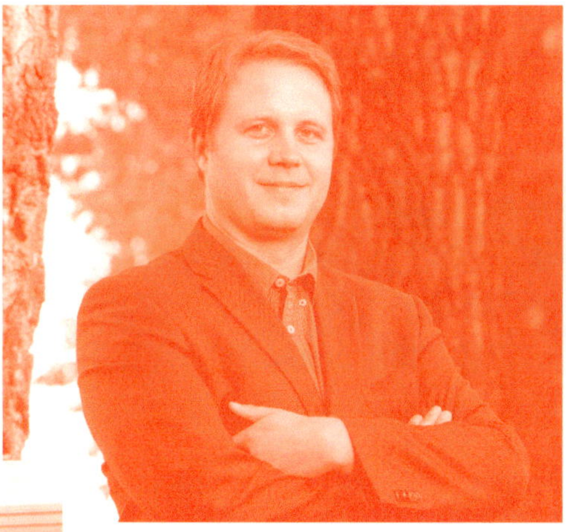

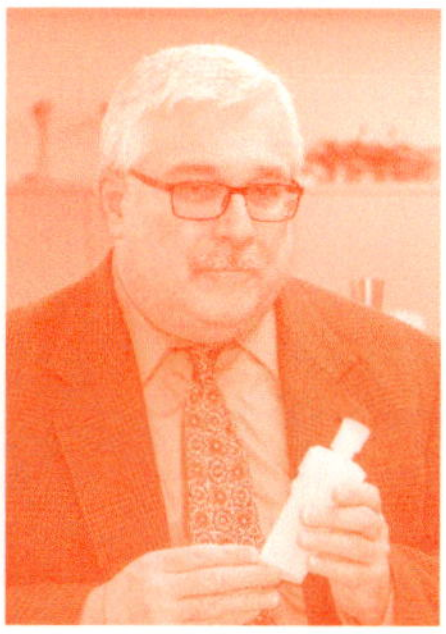

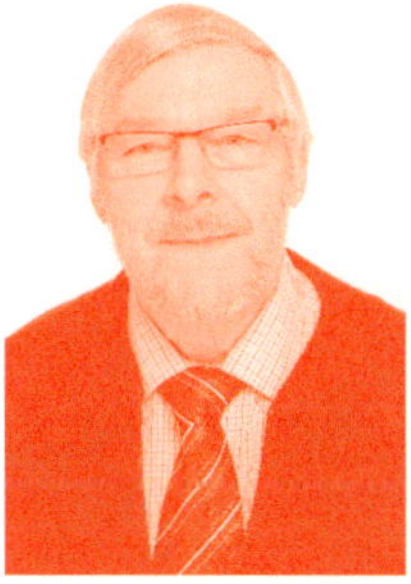

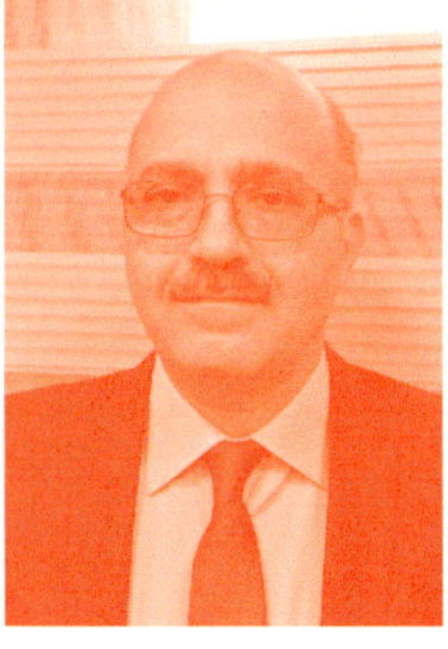

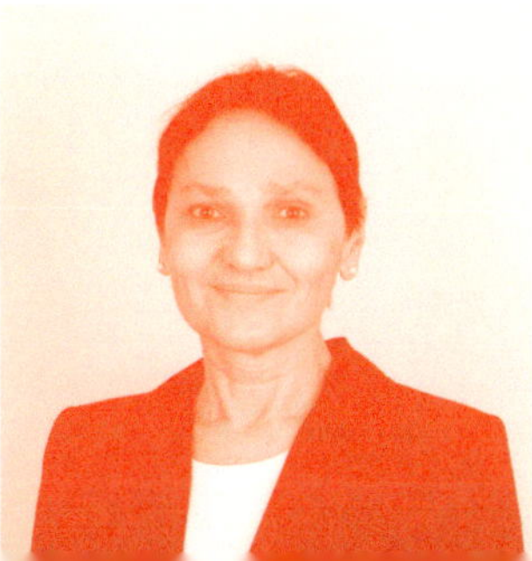

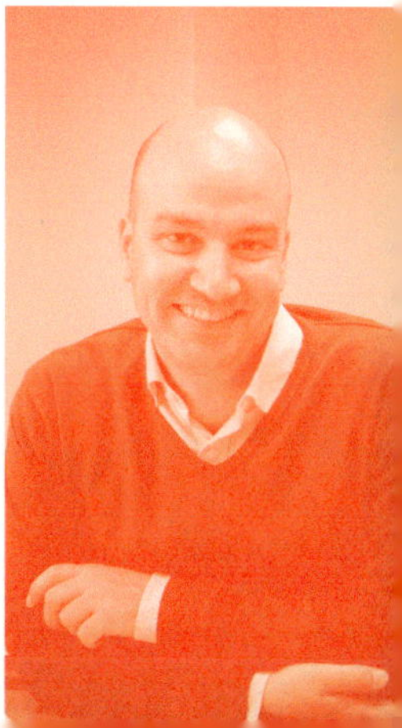

Asthma - Biological Evidences
http://dx.doi.org/10.5772/intechopen.80155
Edited by Celso Pereira

Contributors
Constantine Saadeh, Nicole Davey-Ranasinghe, Wenchao Tang, Kewal Asosingh, Andrew Reichard, Bushra Mubarak, Huma Shakoor, Fozia Masood, Poonam Arora, S. H. Ansari, Samuel N. Nkachukwu Uwaezuoke, Joy N. Eze, Xiaoyan Dong, Nanbert Zhong, Mirjana Turkalj, Ivana Banić, Marzie Zilaee, Seyed Ahmad Hosseini

First published in London, United Kingdom, 2019 by IntechOpen
IntechOpen is the global imprint of INTECHOPEN LIMITED, registered in England and Wales, registration number: 11086078, The Shard, 25th floor, 32 London Bridge Street
London, SE19SG - United Kingdom
Printed in Croatia

British Library Cataloguing-in-Publication Data
A catalogue record for this book is available from the British Library

Additional hard and PDF copies can be obtained from orders@intechopen.com

Asthma - Biological Evidences
Edited by Celso Pereira
p. cm.
Print ISBN 978-1-78984-315-6
Online ISBN 978-1-78984-316-3
eBook (PDF) ISBN 978-1-83962-246-5

For EU product safety concerns:
IN TECH d.o.o., Prolaz Marije Krucifikse Kozulić 3, 51000 Rijeka, Croatia, info@intechopen.com or visit our website at intechopen.com.

Meet the editor

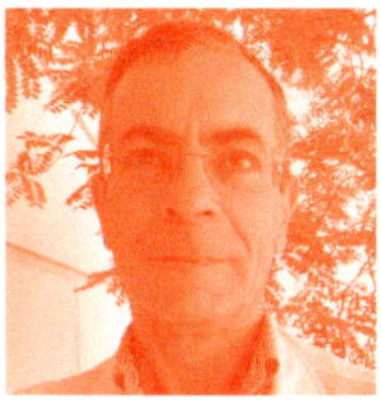

Prof Celso Pereira, MD, PhD, is head-chief of the Clinical Immunology Unit and Clinical Herbal Medicine at the Medicine Faculty of Coimbra University, Portugal. He is a specialist in Immuno-Allergy at Coimbra University's Hospital Centre. He was the past president of the Immuno-Allergy Board of the Portuguese Medical Association. His main activities include clinical practice, education (pre- and post-graduate), and clinical and laboratory research. He is a member of a national committee for vaccination and coordinator of some clinical guidelines approved and under application by Portuguese health authorities. He is also a member of a national committee for diagnostic procedures in the field of allergy and clinical immunology. Dr. Pereira's scientific interests include research in the mechanisms of respiratory allergy, specific immunotherapy, and medicinal herbs.

Contents

Preface

The clinical expression of asthma in its many phenotypes and endotypes is based on multiple and diversified pathogenic mechanisms. Although in the inflammatory process there may be a predominance of some cell lines with very peculiar biological characteristics, there is always a complex and intricate participation of all the elements of the adaptive and innate immune system. Likewise all the resident and structural cells present in the bronchi are active vectors in the chronic inflammation, as are the contiguous extracellular matrix proteins.

Successive genome-wide association studies have proven the polygenic profile of asthma by identifying the complex and extensive networks of critical cellular mediators engaged in local bronchial mucosa as well as regional and systemic inflammation. In this context, a profound knowledge of cell biology is crucial, because it can allow to define a specific pathophysiological way for each clinical phenotype/endotype that may guide to a personalized therapy.

Even though much of the research is currently directed towards new biologics aimed at severe asthma patients, fortunately in clinical practice the overwhelming majority of asthmatics have more favorable treatment options. However, like other chronic inflammatory disorders deficient control is very common in clinical practice, also allying difficulties in adhesion and compliance to a long-lasting treatment plan.

This book exhaustively and didactically covers the biological expression of numerous cells and mediators involved in bronchial inflammation. The authors provide robust information identifying the diversity and complexity of the interrelationships between the different players, drawing attention to critical mechanisms in asthma.

These reviews show the impossibility of standardizing the therapeutic plan for asthma due mainly to the heterogeneity of pathophysiological mechanisms corresponding to different clinical profiles. Asthma, although prevalent in all age groups, is a diverse condition. While in most patients the currently available treatments (different anti-inflammatory drugs and bronchodilators) can help control asthma, they have no effect on other pathways of chronic inflammation, namely those leading to structural changes and remodeling. It is clear that the available biological treatments and others currently in pharmacological trials are clearly insufficient to effectively halt and control inflammation.

This update on the biological aspects of cells and mediators involved in asthma will hopefully open up new lines of research that may lead to new therapeutic approaches to optimize the control of inflammation and other symptoms as well as lung function and patient quality of life. Furthermore, this book highlights the use of new diagnostic procedures in order to identify different asthma biomarkers with high specificity and sensitivity for each predominant pathophysiological mechanism involved. The information contained herein allows for the creation of personalized and effective treatment for asthmatic patients.

Celso Pereira, MD, PhD
Clinical Immunology,
Faculty of Medicine,
University of Coimbra,
Coimbra, Portugal

Chapter 1

Childhood and Adult Asthma: Phenotype- and Endotype-Based Biomarkers

Joy N. Eze and Samuel N. Uwaezuoke

Abstract

The concept of asthma has changed from that of a single disease entity to that of a heterogeneous disease comprising several phenotypes linked to specific endotypes. Recently, significant progress has been made in disease classification into phenotypes and biologically distinct variants (endotypes). Classification of patients into endotypes has led to precision medicine in which specific biomarkers and appropriate individualized treatments have now been identified. Despite the ongoing classification of disease endotypes, the presence or absence of a T-helper 2 (Th2) molecular signature has resulted in the association of asthma endotypes with phenotypes so as to establish responders and non-responders to inhaled corticosteroid therapy. More importantly, biologic therapies predicated on disease endotypes may in future constitute a paradigm shift from the traditional pharmacologic treatments and lead to better prognosis in moderate-to-severe forms of the disease (in which they are presently used). This book chapter aims to discuss the current concepts on asthma classification and biomarker-based diagnosis.

Keywords: asthma, biomarkers, endotypes, heterogeneous disease, phenotypes

1. Introduction

Asthma represents one of the major childhood noncommunicable respiratory diseases worldwide [1]. Asthma is now seen as a complex heterogeneous disease with variable natural history, severity, comorbidities, and therapeutic response. The disease is thus defined in several ways. For instance, asthma is defined as an airway disorder with underlying chronic inflammation characterized by hyper-responsive airway, which results in nonspecific symptoms like recurrent wheezing, breathlessness, nocturnal or early morning cough, and chest tightness. The symptoms tend to change over time and intensity, in conjunction with variable airflow limitation [2]. The disease also represents a syndrome with several phenotypes (the observable physical characteristics from the gene–environment interactions) and endotypes [3]. Research within the last decade has sought to better understand the heterogeneous nature of asthma. Disease heterogeneity particularly manifests in the clinical features, as well as the type and degree of airway inflammation and remodeling. Thus, there is now a paradigm shift in the concept of asthma as a single disease entity to that of a complex cluster of disease phenotypes [4]. Various subtypes of inflammation and complex immunoregulatory pathways and the factors responsible for their failure have now been documented.

2. Asthma phenotypes and endotypes: A snapshot

An endotype is a subtype of a disease recognized by a characteristic pathophysiologic mechanism, whereas a disease phenotype refers to any identifiable characteristic without any evidence of a mechanism [5]. Recent advances in asthma management have tried to group patients by a plethora of possible phenotypic features including age of onset, presence of atopy, airway inflammation and severity of airway obstruction, and the need for drugs. On the basis of the diverse cellular and molecular mechanisms, several phenotypes are currently recognized [6]. Using sputum cytological examination, there is now a classification of the major inflammatory phenotypes into eosinophilic, neutrophilic, mixed-complex inflammation, and pauci-granulocytic phenotypes [7]. Other recognizable phenotypes include early-onset mild allergic asthma, late-onset asthma associated with obesity, and severe nonatopic asthma with frequent exacerbations [8]. Experts from the European Academy of Allergy and Clinical Immunology and the American Academy of Allergy, Asthma, and Immunology produced the PRACTALL (Practical Allergy) consensus report which proposed the use of parameters such as clinical features, biomarkers, pulmonary physiology, genetics, histopathology, therapeutic response, and epidemiology for characterizing disease endotypes [9]. The consensus of opinion was that each endotype should meet at least five of these seven criteria [9].

3. Phenotype- and endotype-based biomarkers

Biomarkers are unique parameters linked to disease endotypes which are estimated for the evaluation of any biologic or pathogenic processes, including responses to therapeutic interventions [5]. Their use has made it possible for novel diagnostic tools and targeted therapies to be developed.

3.1 Phenotype-based inflammatory biomarkers

Several biomarkers are now veritable sources of information with respect to disease phenotypes and therapeutic responses. The major examples are described as follows:

3.1.1 Inflammatory cells

Marked blood eosinophilia has been linked to a severe form of late-onset asthma. In fact, blood or sputum eosinophilia is an indicator of Th2-type inflammation in the lungs, while sputum eosinophilia is associated with exacerbations [10, 11] and airway remodeling in asthma [12, 13]. The actions of T-helper 2 (Th2) cells are believed to trigger the stimulation of eosinophilic infiltration into the airways. Eosinophils are made to evolve from an inactive state to a state of increased hyper-responsiveness by priming agents such as these cytokines, interleukin (IL)-3, IL-4, IL-5, and IL-13 [8], and granulocyte-monocyte colony-stimulating factor (GM-CSF) [14]. IL-4 and IL-13 upregulate vascular adhesion molecules and facilitate the migration of eosinophils into tissue sites of inflammation, while IL-5 facilitates differentiation, survival, and chemotaxis of eosinophils [8, 13, 14].

3.1.2 Proteins

While Th2 cytokines can be assayed from bronchial washings, the approach may not be practicable. Proteins emanating from the bronchus which are linked to Th2 airway inflammation are used as surrogate markers for disease phenotype and endotype. Three genes upregulated by Th2 cytokines (IL-13) have been identified, namely,

POSTN, which encodes periostin; CLCA1, which encodes calcium-activated chloride channel regulator 1; and SERPINB2, which encodes serpin peptidase inhibitor, clade B (ovalbumin), member 2 (serpinB2, also known as plasminogen activator inhibitor-2) [13]. Increased levels of these proteins correlate with higher amount of bronchial tissue IL-13 and IL-5 messenger RNA and elevated number of eosinophils and mast cells. Blood levels of periostin have been studied as a surrogate marker for airway eosinophilia and as a method for predicting response to pharmacologic IL-13 blockade with lebrikizumab and anti-IL-13 antibody. The findings of these proteins in subjects with high Th2 also correlate with better response to ICS therapy than Th2-low group. Thus, identification of these proteins is predictive of corticosteroid-responsive asthma.

3.1.3 Epithelial microRNAs

There is a high differential expression of microRNAs (miRNAs) in the airway epithelium of subjects with asthma as compared with healthy controls [15]. MicroRNAs have been identified as regulators of key biologic processes in epithelial cells such as cell proliferation, cell differentiation, and cell death [16, 17]. Woodruff et al. conducted in vitro experimentation with bronchial epithelial cells and observed that IL-13 had obvious effects on bronchial epithelial miRNA expression and that several of these changes underscored the differences between asthma and health that were seen in humans [13]. Subsequent work focused on constant in vivo and in vitro suppression of four members of the miR-34/449 family (miR-34c-5p, miR- 34c-5p, miR-449a, and miR-449b-5p) in asthma and by IL-13, respectively. These data lend credence to the possible biological role of the miR-34/449 family in airway epithelial cells. It is uncertain whether the potential regulation of miRNAs, or others by IL-13, can be an indicator of a high-Th2 asthma endotype. However, miRNAs possess a relatively distinct characteristic which may qualify them as potential biomarkers. In other words, miRNAs can assume forms in extracellular fluids which are resistant to breakdown by RNases and thus can be estimated in sputum, bronchoalveolar lavage fluid, and blood using PCR, microarrays, and sequencing methods [13]. The following proteins, miR-181a, miR- 146a, and miR-146b, are expressed in spleen CD41 T lymphocytes and probably function as proinflammatory agents in an animal model of asthma [18, 19]. Specifically, there was downregulation of miR-375 in IL-13 transgenic mice and its repression in human bronchial (and esophageal) epithelial cells by IL-13 [20]. In addition, miRNA let-7 possesses a complex but proinflammatory activity in an animal model of the disease [21].

3.1.4 Exhaled nitric oxide (FeNO)

There is a moderate correlation between exhaled nitric oxide and bronchial or blood eosinophilia in asthmatics. The enzyme nitric oxide (NO) synthase that produces NO is under direct regulation of IL-13, which is a Th2 cytokine. Elevated FeNO level reflects increased IL-13 activity [22] and indicates the presence of Th2 phenotype. The FeNO is a consistent predictor of a potential steroid responsiveness more than other indices (spirometry, airway hyper-responsiveness to methacholine, bronchodilator response, peak flow variation, etc.) [23].

3.2 Asthma endotypes and associated biomarkers

3.2.1 Allergic asthma

This is a form of persistent asthma which commences in the pediatric-age period. Sensitization to allergens and allergic rhinitis are prominent features. Inhalation of a specific allergen is a stimulus for the acute constriction of bronchial smooth muscles and subsequent infiltration of inflammatory cells, usually followed by a late asthmatic presentation [9]. This condition is believed to be sustained by a Th2-dominant inflammation. Airway eosinophilia is a common feature, and the disease comprises a wide spectrum of disease severities and therapeutic responses. The explorations of IL-4/IL-13 pathway modifiers and the effectiveness of omalizumab in severe allergic asthma underscore the role of IgE and Th2 cells/cytokines in this endotype. Children with asthma predictive indices (API) are susceptible to developing asthma and may or may not include the classic"allergic asthma endotype." The API include presentation with recurrent wheezing episodes (more than three episodes in the first 3 years of life) and at least one of the three major criteria (personal atopic dermatitis, parental asthma, or sensitization to an aeroallergen) or two of the three minor criteria (peripheral eosinophils >4%, wheezing unrelated to the common cold, or sensitization to a food allergen) [24, 25]. Patients who fulfilled these criteria at 3 years of age are clearly at increased risk of manifesting with active asthma symptoms at 6 years of age [9, 25].

3.2.2 Allergic bronchopulmonary mycosis (ABPM)

This condition develops in adults with asthma or in adult/pediatric patients with cystic fibrosis [26]. It is characterized by hypersensitivity reaction to airway colonization by molds, especially *Aspergillus fumigatus* [9, 26]. The main histological feature of ABPM is allergic (eosinophilic) mucin-harboring hyphae in the bronchi, as the induction of the formation of eosinophilic extracellular DNA cell death (ETosis) by viable fungi remains vital [26]. Clinically, ABPM is characterized by episodic bronchial obstruction and mucoid impaction, peripheral blood eosinophilia, elevated serum IgE levels, IgE and IgG antibodies specific for fungi, and typical radiographic findings [9, 26]. A mixed picture of neutrophilic and eosinophilic airway inflammation has also been described [9]. This endotype is characterized by severe bronchial asthma with recurrent exacerbations and progressive lung damage but may respond to systemic glucocorticoids, antifungal agents, and the anti-IgE monoclonal antibody (mAb), omalizumab [9, 26]. Patients develop bronchiectasis and fixed airflow obstruction over time. Early-onset ABPM may be a sequela of the allergic asthma endotype or cystic fibrosis [9].

3.2.3 Aspirin-sensitive asthma (ASA)

It almost always appears in adulthood and has a distinct clinical presentation, presenting after the intake of a nonsteroidal anti-inflammatory drug (NSAID) [9, 27]. Severe and prolonged airway obstruction is characteristically associated with chronic/severe rhinosinusitis and nasal polyps (aspirin-exacerbated respiratory disease), peripheral blood eosinophilia, and raised urinary leukotrienes at baseline and post-aspirin challenge. Pathophysiologically, ASA has been linked to increased elaboration of cysteinyl leukotriene and increased expression of leukotriene C4 synthase. Cysteinyl leukotriene receptor antagonists and leukotriene C4 synthesis inhibitors ameliorate ASA symptoms although these medications do not protect the patient from NSAID adverse effects [28].

A subgroup of individuals with late-onset asthma in adulthood fulfills the criteria for a distinctive asthma endotype. They constitute about 20% of patients grouped as having refractory asthma and exhibit a typical pattern of severe exacerbations which are circumvented by systemic corticosteroid but not ICS, as well as hyper-eosinophilia in the blood (>1000/mm^3) and sputum (>10%) [29]. These patients also have a lower prevalence of atopy than the "allergic asthma" endotype [9]. Moreover, the degrees of bronchodilator responsiveness and nonspecific airway hyper-responsiveness may be less than those in the "allergic asthma" endotype. Studies have suggested that anti-IL-5 therapy may also be effective in this endotype [30, 31].

3.2.4 Cross-country skiers' asthma

It is defined as episodes of asthma symptoms and/or wheeze closely associated with strenuous skiing-related exercise and concomitant airway hyper-responsiveness. An extremely cold, dry climate promotes the evolution of this type of asthma in comparison with warmer, more humid conditions [32, 33]. Cross-country skiers' asthma is rarely associated with allergic sensitization but is characterized by airway inflammation dominated by elevated numbers of lymphocytes, macrophages, and neutrophils but rarely eosinophils. Lymphoid aggregates in the form of bronchus-associated lymphoid tissue in the mucosa, as well as evidence of airway remodeling with thickening of the reticuloepithelial membrane can be identified in bronchoscopic studies.

Amateur endurance runners had an elevated number of bronchial epithelial cells and apoptosis of bronchial cells in induced sputum evolving through repeated half-marathon races, in addition to increased serum levels of CC16 and raised supernatant interleukin (IL)-8 levels in induced sputum [34]. Furthermore, urinary levels of CC16 are increased following exercise [35, 36]. Increased expression as measured by polymerase chain reaction (PCR) of the gel-forming mucin, MUC5AC, in induced sputum and levels of supernatant cysteinyl leukotrienes and higher ratio of cysteinyl leukotrienes to prostaglandins have been reported. This endotype is resistant to ICS therapy, but its symptoms often improve with a drop in intensity of training.

Phenotype	Eosinophilic asthma
	Endotypes: allergic asthma (adult)*, aspirin-sensitive asthma, severe late-onset hyper-eosinophilic asthma*, ABPM*
Phenotype	Exacerbation-prone asthma
	Endotypes: allergic asthma (adult)*, aspirin-sensitive asthma*, late-onset hyper-eosinophilic asthma, API-positive preschool wheezers*, ABPM*, viral-exacerbated asthma, premenstrual asthma
Phenotype	Obesity-related asthma
	Endotypes: airflow obstruction caused by obesity, severe steroid-dependent asthma, severe late-onset hyper-eosinophilic asthma*
Phenotype	Exercise-induced asthma
	Endotypes: cross-country skiers' asthma, other forms of elite-athlete asthma, allergic asthma, API-positive preschool wheezers*
Phenotype	Adult-onset asthma
	Endotypes: aspirin-sensitive asthma*, infection-induced asthma, severe late-onset hyper-eosinophilic asthma*
Phenotype	Fixed airflow limitation
	Endotypes: noneosinophilic (neutrophilic) asthma
Phenotype	Poorly steroid-responsive asthma
	Endotypes: noneosinophilic (neutrophilic) asthma, steroid-insensitive eosinophilic asthma, airflow obstruction caused by obesity

Culled from [9].
**NB: asthma phenotypes can be present in more than 1 endotypes and endotypes can contain more than 1 phenotype.*

Table 1.
Proposed relationship between asthma phenotypes and endotypes.

Endotypes	Biomarkers
Asthma predictive index preschool wheezers	>4% eosinophil in blood (minor), aeroallergen-specific IgE
Allergic asthma (adults)	Positive SPT, elevated IgE/elevated FeNO
Severe late-onset hyper-eosinophilic asthma	Peripheral blood eosinophilia
Allergic bronchopulmonary mycosis (ABPM)	Blood eosinophilia, markedly elevated IgE and specific IgE
Aspirin-sensitive asthma	Blood eosinophilia, increased urinary LTEs
Cross-country skiers' asthma	FeNO normal, normal blood eosinophil count, increased urinary LTEs

SPT, skin prick test; FeNO, fractional exhaled nitric oxide; IgE, immunoglobulin E; LTEs, leukotrienes.

Table 2.
Biomarkers associated with some endotypes.

Obviously, the pathophysiologic mechanisms underlying the various asthma phenotypes and endotypes are diverse. Thus, the biomarkers of these phenotypes and endotypes are different but may be interwoven since phenotypes may be linked with more than one endotype and vice versa. **Table 1** shows the possible relationship between asthma phenotypes and endotypes, while **Table 2** shows some of the biomarkers associated with disease endotypes.

4. Conclusion

The pathogenic concept of asthma in childhood and adulthood is changing. Its current concept is that of a heterogeneous and genetically complex disease with several phenotypes presenting with distinct clinical features which are linked to endotypes with different underlying mechanisms and characteristic therapeutic responses. More importantly, the categorization of endotypes in childhood asthma is still evolving as disease classification has now been able to associate phenotypes with endotypes based on airway and serum biomarkers. Better still, there is a potential nexus between disease phenotypes and endotypes or biomarkers, as well as some potential personalized therapeutic options. In the future, endotypes may be used together with specific biomarkers to predict responses to targeted treatments.

Author details

Joy N. Eze[1,2] and Samuel N. Uwaezuoke[1,2*]

1 College of Medicine, University of Nigeria, Enugu, Nigeria

2 University of Nigeria Teaching Hospital, Enugu, Nigeria

*Address all correspondence to: samuel.uwaezuoke@unn.edu.ng

References

[1] Asher I, Pearce N. Global burden of asthma among children. The International Journal of Tuberculosis and Lung Disease. 2014;**18**(11): 1269-1278. DOI: 10.5588/ijtld.14.0170

[2] Bateman ED, Hurd SS, Barnes PJ, et al. Global strategy for asthma management and prevention: GINA executive summary. The European Respiratory Journal. 2008;**31**(1):143-178. DOI: 10.1183/09031936.00138707

[3] Lockey RF. Asthma phenotypes: An approach to the diagnosis and treatment of asthma. The Journal of Allergy and Clinical Immunology. 2014;**2**(6): 682-685. DOI: 10.1016/j.jaip.2014.09.008

[4] Bierbaum S, Heinzmann A. The genetics of bronchial asthma in children. Respiratory Medicine. 2007;**101**:1369-1375. DOI: 10.1016/j.rmed.2007.01.018

[5] Agache I, Akdis CA. Endotypes of allergic diseases and asthma: An important step in building blocks for the future of precision medicine. Allergology International. 2016;**65**: 243-252. DOI: 10.1016/j.alit.2016.04.011

[6] Papi A, Brightling C, Pedersen SE, Reddel HK. Asthma. Lancet. 2018;**391**(10122):783-800. DOI: 10.1016/S0140-6736(17)33311-1

[7] Simpson JL, Scott R, Boyle MJ, Gibson PG. Inflammatory subtypes in asthma: Assessment and identification using induced sputum. Respirology. 2006;**11**(1):54-61. DOI: 10.1111/j.1440-1843.2006.00784.x

[8] Corren J. Asthma phenotype and endotypes: An evolving paradigm for classification. Discovery Medicine. 2013;**15**(83):243-249

[9] Lötvall J, Akdis CA, Bacharier LB, et al. Asthma endotypes: A new approach to classification of disease entities within the asthma syndrome. The Journal of Allergy and Clinical Immunology. 2011;**127**(2):355-360. DOI: 10.1016/j.jaci.2010.11.037

[10] Casciano J, Krishnan JA, Small MB, et al. Burden of asthma with elevated blood eosinophil levels. BMC Pulmonary Medicine. 2016;**16**(1):100. DOI: 10.1186/s12890-016-0263-8

[11] Casciano J, Krishnan J, Dotiwala Z, Li C, Sun SX. Clinical and economic burden of elevated blood eosinophils in patients with and without uncontrolled asthma. Journal of Managed Care & Specialty Pharmacy. 2017;**23**(1):85-91. DOI: 10.18553/jmcp.2017.23.1.85

[12] Bergeron C, Tulic MK, Hamid Q. Airway remodeling in asthma: From bench side to clinical practice. Canadian Respiratory Journal. 2010;**17**(4):e85-e94. DOI: 10.1155/2010/318029

[13] Woodruff PG. Subtypes of asthma defined by epithelial cell expression of messenger RNA and MicroRNA. Annals of the American Thoracic Society. 2013;**10**(Suppl):S186-S189. DOI: 10.1513/AnnalsATS.201303-070AW

[14] George L, Brightling CE. Eosinophilic airway inflammation: Role in asthma and chronic obstructive pulmonary disease. Therapeutic Advances in Chronic Disease. 2016;**7**(1):34-51. DOI: 10.1177/2040622315609251

[15] Solberg OD, Ostrin EJ, Love MI, et al. Airway epithelial miRNA expression is altered in asthma. American Journal of Respiratory and Critical Care Medicine. 2012;**186**(10):965-974. DOI: 10.1164/rccm.201201-0027OC

[16] Corney DC, Flesken-Nikitin A, Godwin AK, Wang W, Nikitin AY.

MicroRNA-34b and MicroRNA-34c are targets of p53 and cooperate in control of cell proliferation and adhesion-independent growth. Cancer Research. 2007;**67**(18):8433-8438. DOI: 10.1158/0008-5472.CAN-07-1585

[17] Liu X, Nelson A, Wang X, et al. MicroRNA-146a modulates human bronchial epithelial cell survival in response to the cytokine-induced apoptosis. Biochemical and Biophysical Research Communications. 2009;**380**(1):177-182. DOI: 10.1016/j.bbrc.2009.01.066

[18] Simpson LJ, Patel S, Bhakta NR, et al. A miRNA upregulated in asthma airway T cells promotes T H 2 cytokine production HHS public access. Nature Immunology. 2014;**15**(12):1162-1170. DOI: 10.1038/ni.3026

[19] Liu Y, Chen Z, Xu K, et al. Next generation sequencing for miRNA profile of spleen CD4 + T cells in the murine model of acute asthma. Epigenomics. 2018;**10**(8):1071-1083. DOI: doi.org/10.2217/epi-2018-0043

[20] Lu TX, Lim E-J, Wen T, et al. MiR-375 is down-regulated in epithelial cells after IL-13 stimulation and regulates an IL-13 induced epithelial transcriptome. Mucosal Immunology. 2012;**5**(4):388-396. DOI: 10.1038/mi.2012.16

[21] Polikepahad S, Knight JM, Naghavi AO, et al. Proinflammatory role for let-7 MicroRNAs in experimental asthma. The Journal of Biological Chemistry. 2010;**285**(39):30139-30149. DOI: 10.1074/jbc.M110.145698

[22] Chibana K, Trudeau JB. Mustovitch, et al. IL-13 induced increases in nitrite levels are primarily driven by increases in inducible nitric oxide synthase as compared with effects on arginases in human primary bronchial epithelial cells. Clinical and Experimental Allergy. 2008;**38**(6):936-946. DOI: 10.1111/j.1365-2222.2008.02969.x

[23] Cowan DC, Cowan JO, Palmay R, Williamson A, Taylor R. Effects of steroid therapy on inflammatory cell subtypes in asthma. Thorax. 2010;**65**(5):384-390. DOI: 10.1136/thx.2009.126722

[24] Castro-Rodríguez JA, Holberg CJ, Wright AL, Martinez FD. A clinical index to define risk of asthma in young children with recurrent wheezing. American Journal of Respiratory and Critical Care Medicine. 2000;**162**:1403-1406. DOI: doi.org/10.1164/ajrccm.162.4.9912111

[25] Castro-Rodriguez JA, Santiago P. The asthma predictive index: A very useful tool for predicting asthma in young children. The Journal of Allergy and Clinical Immunology. 2010;**126**:212-216

[26] Asano K, Kamei K, Hebisawa A. Allergic bronchopulmonary mycosis—Pathophysiology, histology, diagnosis, and treatment. Asia Pacific Allergy. 2018;**8**(3):e24. DOI: 10.5415/apallergy.2018.8.e24

[27] Morwood K, Gillis D, Smith W, Kette F. Aspirin-sensitive asthma. Internal Medicine Journal. 2005;**35**(4):240-246. DOI: doi.org/10.1111/j.1445-5994.2004.00801.x

[28] Dahlén B, Nizankowska E, Szczeklik A, et al. Benefits from adding the 5-lipoxygenase inhibitor zileuton to conventional therapy in aspirin-intolerant asthmatics. American Journal of Respiratory and Critical Care Medicine. 1998;**157**(4 Pt 1):1187-1194. DOI: 10.1164/ajrccm.157.4.9707089

[29] Haldar P, Pavord ID, Shaw DE, et al. Cluster analysis and clinical asthma phenotypes. American Journal of Respiratory and Critical Care Medicine. 2008;**178**(3):218-224

[30] Nair P, Pizzichini MMM, Kjarsgaard M, et al. Mepolizumab for

prednisone-dependent asthma with sputum eosinophilia. The New England Journal of Medicine. 2009;**360**(10): 985-993. DOI: 10.1056/NEJMoa0805435

[31] Nair P, O'Byrne PM. Measuring Eosinophils to make treatment decisions in asthma. Chest. 2016;**150**(3):485-487. DOI: doi.org/10.1016/j.chest.2016.07.009

[32] Carlsen KH. Mechanisms of asthma development in elite athletes. Breathe. 2012;**8**(4):279-284. DOI: 10.1183/20734735.009512

[33] Carlsen KH, Lødrup-Carlsen KC. Asthma and the Olympics. The Journal of Allergy and Clinical Immunology. 2016;**138**(2):409-410

[34] Chimenti L, Morici G, Paternò A, et al. Bronchial epithelial damage after a half-marathon in nonasthmatic amateur runners. American Journal of Physiology. Lung Cellular and Molecular Physiology. 2010;**298**:857-862. DOI: 10.1152/ajplung.00053.2010

[35] Bolger C, Tufvesson E, Anderson SD, et al. Effect of inspired air conditions on exercise-induced bronchoconstriction and urinary CC16 levels in athletes. Journal of Applied Physiology. 2011;**111**:1059-1065. DOI: 10.1152/japplphysiol.00113.2011

[36] Bolger C, Tufvesson E, Sue-Chu M, et al. Hyperpnoea-induced bronchoconstriction and urinary CC16 levels in athletes. Medicine and Science in Sports and Exercise. 2011;**43**(7):1207-1213. DOI: 10.1249/MSS.0b013e31820750d8

Chapter 2

Clinical Applications of Impulse Oscillometry

Constantine Saadeh and Nicole Davey-Ranasinghe

Abstract

Impulse oscillometry is a noninvasive procedure that can be performed within few minutes. The purpose of the procedure is to measure the resistance of the small and large airways, as well as the reactants of the airways. It is gradually gaining popularity in evaluating lung function, particularly in patients with asthma and COPD. In contrast to spirometry, the test performs measurement during tidal breathing. In other words, forced exhalation is not required. Other advantages include, but are not limited to, evaluating COPD patients' reversibility which is rarely noted on spirometry. IOS also is tool for chronic management of patients with asthma and COPD while on treatment. It can evaluate children with asthma even as young as 2 years old. Spirometry requires the child to cooperate and usually is of meaningful use beginning at the age of 5 years old. Other potential applications include early evaluation of transplant rejection, cystic fibrosis, and vocal cord disorder. In this chapter, we will explore the procedure itself, the settings, advantages and disadvantages, and comparative data with spirometry.

Keywords: impulse oscillometry, spirometry, asthma, COPD

1. Introduction

The expert panel 3 of the National Asthma Education and Prevention Program defines asthma as "a common chronic disorder of the airways that is complex and characterized by variable and recurring symptoms, airflow obstruction, bronchial hyperresponsiveness, and an underlying inflammation. The interaction of these features of asthma determines the clinical manifestations and severity of asthma and the response to treatment." This definition allows for incorporation of the clinical, physiological, and pathological findings of asthma. Traditional spirometry, while the gold standard, can be unreliable in pediatric patients and is dependent on patient effort. Impulse oscillometry is a clinical tool that is independent of patient effort and allows for diagnosis and management of pediatric and adult patients with asthma. IOS can enhance the clinical evaluation for patients with asthma. IOS is a technique that measures airway impedance (resistance and reactance). IOS is a noninvasive technique that is beneficial either as a single modality or in combination with traditional spirometry for patients in the diagnosis and management of asthma.

2. Overview

Impulse oscillometry or IOS is a measure of both small and large airway resistance. In addition, resonance capacitance or reactance is also obtained via impulse spirometry. It is also referred to as forced oscillation since impulses are sent at periodic intervals into the airways. The measurement of airway resistance and reactance is performed in a noninvasive, relatively independent, and minimally intrusive manner during spontaneous tidal breathing [1].

In contrast to traditional spirometry, impulse oscillometry or IOS tracing is independent of age, height, weight, or gender in adolescents or adults 13 years or older. In other words, normal values are the same whether the patient is 13 or 60 years old. The most relevant findings include R5, R15 or higher, and AX. R5 reflects the small airway resistance. However, R5 is the summation of small and large airways. R15 or higher signifies only the larger airways. AX is low-frequency integrated impedance reactance at R5 and is referred to as purely reactance.

In this chapter, we will review briefly the IOS procedure. We will then guide the reader to the useful applications of this methodology and the diagnosis and follow-up in patients with asthma in terms of actual diagnosis, follow-up with treatment as outpatient, and documentation of response to treatment. Response to treatment can be gauged via handheld nebulizer treatment in the acute setting. In addition, treatment with inhaled corticosteroids or inhaled corticosteroid/LABA or long-acting beta agonists has also been observed independent of spirometry [2]. We will also review the literature regarding the comparison of this modality to traditional spirometry. Finally, we will briefly outline future directions in the evaluation of other respiratory disorders.

3. Impulse oscillometry

3.1 Technique

The technique of IOS is effort independent. However, it does require breathing through the mouth as noted below. The IOS technique was performed as previously described. Briefly, patients are seated comfortably in a no swivel chair (**Figure 1**).

Nose clips were applied, and a special mouthpiece was used. For IOS measurements, patients may be advised to cradle their cheeks with their hands. Patients are allowed to breathe normally while the loudspeaker delivered intermittent

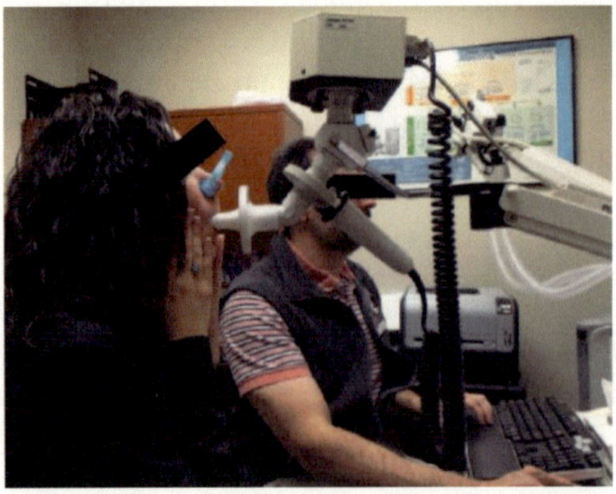

Figure 1.
The subject during tidal breathing inhales and exhale in a closed system. Technician is watching the screen for the sinusoidal waves to pick up the best reading.

multi-frequency impulses over a minimum of a 30-s period. A trained technician will be guiding and assisting the patient during the procedure, which involves three to five sinusoidal readings, depending on the incidence of cough, swallowing, and holding of breath. The recordings with the best coherence at frequencies from 5 to 30 Hz were chosen. The technician was also trained to capture subclinical leaks through the mouthpiece, and leaky recordings were discarded. The pre- and post-bronchodilator assessments took at least 10 min and used ultrasonic nebulizer. The IOS parameters measured were R5, R15, and AX.

Traditionally, spirometry is utilized to evaluate lung function in both children and adults. There is no doubt that spirometry is of greater utility at least for most practitioners who diagnose and manage asthma. However, the limitations include difficulty conducting the measurement in patients who are less than 5 years old. Even in patients who are 5 years old and older, the predicted FEV1 may not be as accurate as it is in adults. On the other hand, IOS is more feasible in terms of detecting small airway dysfunction [27, 28]. Classically, small airway dysfunction is detected via the FEF 25/FEF 75. This is highly volume dependent as patients may be unable to perform a complete expiratory maneuver from total lung capacity to residual volume.

Even in adults, spirometry itself has its own limitations. FEV1 or the forced expiration volume in the first second is dependent on the ability of the patient to take a deep breath and forcefully exhale until the residual volume is reached. The FEV1 is then compared to a predicted value which is determined via statistical analysis of normal people. Therefore, patients who participate in athletics, for example, may have a higher FEV1 than the predicted value. However, these patients may also have abnormal IOS even though they have supernormal FEV1. In addition, patients with lower predicted value may show improvement in the IOS even though the spirometry may not change. The improvement can be noted acutely via handheld nebulizer or chronically through the use of maintenance inhalers such as corticosteroids.

4. Measurements

Impulse oscillometry in contrast to spirometry measures the resistance and the airways as well as the reactants. The resistance in the airways is referred to as R5 which is the resistance in the small airways. R15 or higher is a measurement of the resistance in the larger airways. It is important to note that the resistance in the small airways or R5 is the summation of the small and large airways, and therefore the difference between R5 and R15 or higher is the actual small airway measurement. The integrated impedance reactants at R5 or above are referred to as AX. AX is considered the area under the X curve from the beginning of normal inspiration. The reactants are a more sensitive guideline for patient evaluation and asthma. A normal AX is 3 cm of water or less in children who are 13 years and older throughout adulthood. Children who are 5 years or younger have poor lung compliance. Therefore, a normal AX in this age group varies, but usually it is 30 cm of water or less. Therefore, in the younger age group since there is variation in the measurement of AX, it is reasonable to always measure the AX pre-and post-bronchodilation with short-acting beta agonist. This will give better determination of the actual pulmonary status of the patient. As a result of that, children who are between the ages of 6 and 12 will have an AX in between 30 and 3 cm of water. In this group of patients, it is important to follow up these patients not only with measurement of reactance or AX at baseline but also to check that nebulizer treatment is followed with short-acting beta. These patients were on rather than of equal or less of 1000 μg per day at least 2 weeks after treatment with inhaled maintenance corticosteroids or combination. The combination in general will be inhaled corticosteroids with long-acting beta agonist **Figure 3**.

The trained technician will be able to choose the recordings with the best coherence at frequencies between 5 and 30 Hz. The ideal coherence should be 0.9, 1, 1, 1 at 5, 10, 15, and 20 Hz, respectively. The technician is also trained to capture subclinical leaks through the mouthpiece, and leak recordings should be discarded.

5. Role of IOS in asthma

Published observations by the author and colleagues have shown that patients with asthma showed improvement in the IOS values. This has been observed through the measurement of the reactance or AX immediately following nebulizer treatment as well as definite improvement 3 months or more after the start of inhaled corticosteroids or a combination of inhaled corticosteroids with long-acting beta agonist. The FEV1 in these patients showed improvement in the minority of patients, while the reactance or AX improved in all the patients who were tested. There were 39 patients who were adults in this age group. **Figure 1** above shows in office IOS. **Figures 2** and **3** below revels the improvement in IOS immediately following nebulizer treatment and 3 months later in an individual patient [26–28].

The role of small airway dysfunction in adults with asthma has been demonstrated in at least 31–47% of 196 patients who were diagnosed with asthma and had insufficient control of their symptoms. Twenty percent of these patients had poorly controlled asthma. Irrespective of their smoking history, both impulse oscillometry and nitric oxide measurements in the exhaled breath or FENO were more sensitive

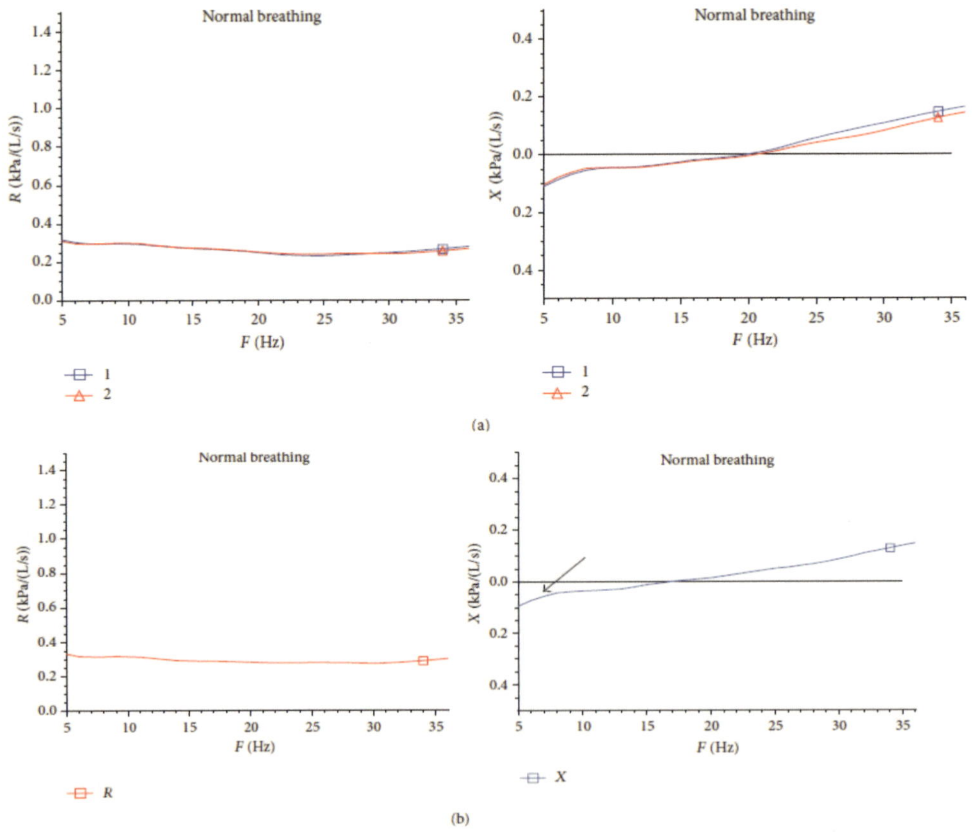

Figure 2.
(a) Patient 15 before bronchodilator. (b) Patient after bronchodilator.

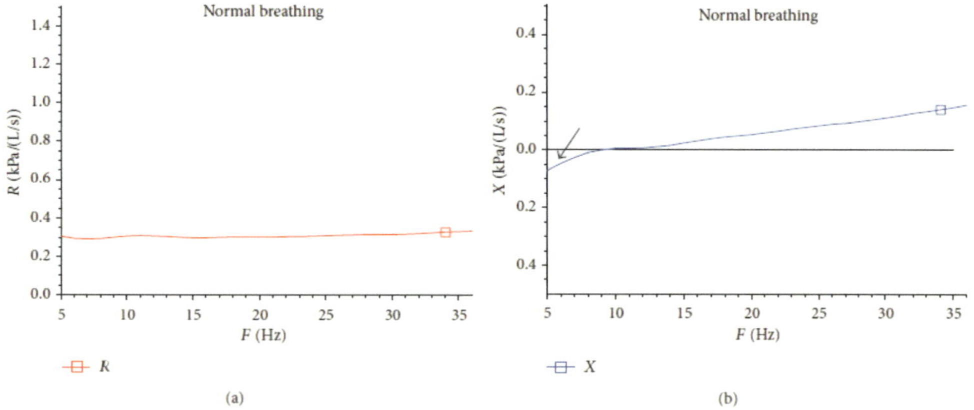

Figure 3.
Patient 15 follow-up (post) (shadowed area AX). Notice normal resistance (a) and normal AX (b) following inhaled corticosteroids for at least two weeks.

in predicting small airway dysfunction than traditional spirometric measurements. The authors concluded that even though nitric oxide measurement was slightly more sensitive than IOS, both of these tests were complimentary in determining the severity of peripheral airway dysfunction. However, in this study, the risk factors for peripheral airway dysfunction were noted to be in patients who have traditionally positive smoking history, elevated blood eosinophils, and dose with low baseline FEV1. Nevertheless, the role of impulse oscillometry in this study should be strongly emphasized (**Figure 3**) [3].

In children with asthma, IOS was noted to be more useful than spirometry and identifying both the asthma and predicting loss of control and exacerbations. This can help with early intervention when the spirometry is normal, but the IOS is showing abnormality. In particular, children are known to have more peripheral or small airway dysfunction. Traditionally this has been dependent upon forced expiration flow between 25 and 75%. Recent studies have shown that IOS is a better predictor particularly in measurement of the small airways or R5 as well as the reactance or AX in the initial evaluation and response to treatment. IOS had improved diagnostic capability in identifying patients with uncontrolled asthma during select baseline values. In the longitudinal analysis of 54 children between the ages of 7 and 17 years old with mild to moderate asthma, both R5 and AX showed inadequate control of asthma 8–12 weeks after the initial visit than spirometric measurements. This included FEF 25–75%. Scholz and colleagues evaluated the value of IOS compared with spirometry and methacholine challenge as predictors of asthma exacerbation in children who are 4–7 years old during 1-year observation. R5 was more predictive of an exacerbation even at the time when the patient was not having any symptoms. The FEV1 or FEV1/FVC and methacholine challenge via spirometry were also normal in these children. In preschool children, normal IOS findings in children between the ages of 2 and 7 years old in patients with asthma are unlikely to have decreased lung function in adolescence based on their initial IOS measurements [4, 5].

Small airways of the lung are defined as the bronchial passages that are less than 2 mm in diameter. They are located beyond the seventh or eighth generation of the tracheobronchial tree. These airways account for more than 90% of the cross-sectional area of the lung and terminate with the alveolar sacs [6].

The small airways have no cartilage to support the structure and are therefore more easily collapsible upon compression. Small airway disease affects the majority of asthmatics across the spectrum of severity. The production of small particle inhaled corticosteroids has enhanced the delivery of inhaled corticosteroids to the smaller airways. This certainly has improved lung function in both adults and children with asthma. Traditionally, high-resolution CT of the chest has been a noninvasive direct radiographic assessment of the luminal caliber and wall thickness of the medium and large airways that are more than 2 mm in diameter. However, this modality has difficulty in evaluating airways that are less than 2 mm in diameter. About 5–10% of patients with asthma are deemed to have severe disease as defined by the European Respiratory Society and the American Thoracic Society as asthma that requires treatment with high-dose inhaled corticosteroids plus a second controller and/or systemic corticosteroids to prevent it from becoming uncontrolled or that remains uncontrolled despite this therapy. Treatment compliance such as appropriate use of inhalers is essential for disease management [7]. Even though there is no gold standard technique for the assessment or diagnosis of small airway, impulse oscillometry in particular has been shown to be effective in the evaluation of small airways either alone or in a combination with exhaled nitric oxide measurement [8].

6. IOS and airway hyperreactivity

The role of IOS in bronchial challenge has also been studied. Bronchial challenge test with methacholine or histamine directly or indirectly such as mannitol may be used in every day clinical practice to identify the presence of airway hyperactivity. Airway hyperactivity is the hallmark of persistent asthma. It is particularly useful when the diagnosis of asthma is in doubt such as patients who are experiencing unexplained cough with normal spirometry. Theoretically, performing IOS with normal tidal breathing is much easier for patients to perform with repeated measurements during challenge. Bronchial irritation such as coughing may pose some limitation while performing the test with spirometry. Eighteen adult patients with mild to moderate persistent asthma had methacholine and histamine challenges measuring both spirometry and IOS. A decrease in the FEV1 by 20% was almost equivalent to a 37% drop in R5 for methacholine and 35% decrease for R5 with histamine. The authors concluded that 40% decrease in R5 may be justifiable to approximately extrapolate to the drop in the FEV1 by 20% for both methacholine and histamine challenge [9, 10]. Similar values on R5 or AX were noted in another study. Improvement by 40% or more on the AX value may carry the same significance as a drop in the FEV1 by 20% without the risk of irritation through forced exhalation. Studies in children are very limited in this regard. One study has noted that in children between the ages of 3 and 8 years old, a change in the R5/R20 after methacholine challenge was significantly higher in those children with more severe asthma as shown by increased exercise-induced bronchospasm and short-acting beta 2 agonist use [11].

In another study, 48 young children with asthma undergoing methacholine challenge noted that a drop of 45% in R5 had the equivalents of a drop in the FEV1 by 20%. In addition, significant increase in resistance was seen well before a change in the FEV1 at lower methacholine dosages suggesting that IOS is more sensitive than spirometry [12].

Hyperresponsiveness was also studied in patients with mild to moderate adult asthma. Patients were recruited between the ages of 18 and 65 years old. FEV1 was noted to be greater than 80% of what is predicted in these patients. Diurnal FEV1 variation was less than 30%. These patients were on equal or less of 1000 mcg/day of beclomethasone dipropionate or equivalent dose. These patients were recruited prospectively. Bronchial challenge was performed with inhaled methacholine and histamine. Twenty-one participants were randomized. Eighteen of whom, ten women and eight men, completed the protocol. All of these patients were used in this analysis, and the mean age was 36 years old. The PC 20 over the FEV1 dropped by 20% following the challenge was noted at equivalents of 43.5% drop in R5 and the methacholine challenge, while it was 45% on the histamine challenge. The magnitude of change seen was greater for all IOS indices including R5 and R5–R20 area under the curve as well as what is referred to as resident frequency or X5. X5 correlated well with the AX. The significance of this study is that these patients were identified as having mild to moderate adult asthma. These patients were well controlled with inhaled corticosteroids. Therefore, they had normal FEV1 at baseline. This study correlated with what has been reported in the literature regarding the application of IOS in SSA and hyperactivity in patients with asthma [13].

In terms of bronchial hyperresponsiveness, cough is an important consideration. Cough is a complex reflex that typically acts as a valuable protective airway clearance mechanism. It arises from irritation of the intrapulmonary and extrapulmonary airways. When the cough reflex is activated, there is an initial inspiratory phase followed by the glottic closure. There is prompt increase in intrathoracic pressure. This is followed by forced expiration and the opening of the glottis. As a result, gas is expired at a high flow rate along with the characteristic audible sound recognized as cough. Patients with asthma or chronic cough and suspected cough-variant asthma participated in a prospective study. The purpose of the study was to compare the bronchodilating effect of deep inspiration in patients with chronic asthma, cough-variant asthma, and chronic cough using high dose of methacholine. These were patients who are between the ages of 18 and 65. Twenty-eight patients out of 56 that were screened were included in the study. Fifteen of these patients were taking inhaled corticosteroids, and nine were taking long-acting beta agonist. The total resistance did not differ significantly on any of these 3 groups. However, small airway resistance or R5 worsened in patients with cough-variant asthma and chronic asthma but did not with chronic cough. Similar findings were noted with spirometry. The purpose of the study was to show that deep inspiration can reverse the obstructive effect due to airway closure but not the obstruction due to large airway narrowing. However, as a secondary finding, impulse oscillometry reproduces the same results as spirometry with methacholine challenge with more comfort during the study. This correlated with the other findings as noted above [14].

7. IOS and pro-inflammatory mediators

Asthma is considered a chronic respiratory disease characterized by airway inflammation. Airway inflammation can lead to airway remodeling and hyperresponsiveness. Airway remodeling refers to the structural changes in the airway including but not limited to the airway smooth muscle, airway epithelia, blood vessels, as well as the extracellular matrix. This can manifest itself as an increase in the airway smooth muscle mass, epithelial injury, epithelial cell hyperplasia, goblet cell hyperplasia, thickening of the basement membrane, and angiogenesis. The mechanism of airway remodeling is still unclear. It is noted that multiple cytokines, chemokines, and transcription factors as well as growth factors are released from inflammatory cells. Structural cells are also involved in the airway remodeling. For example, TGF-beta and vascular endothelial growth factor or VEGF are released by the structural cells.

Follistatin-like protein 1 or FSTL1 is also known as transforming growth factor-beta 1-stimulated clone 36. It is a secreted glycoprotein of 308 amino acids. The function of FSTL1 is not completely understood. It has been shown to play a key role in tumor propagation and bone metastasis, chronic pain hypersensitivity, inflammation and insulin resistance, and obesity and regulation of erythropoiesis as well as physical development. Several studies have shown that FSTL1 may play an important role in the respiratory system. It is important in lung development, cartilage formation, and alveolar maturation. No count of FSTL1 and mice is embryonic clear lethal, and these mice display multiple developmental abnormalities of the respiratory and skeletal systems. In a recent study, 32 asthmatics and 25 controls were enrolled for routine blood testing. Spirometry and impulse oscillometry were performed. Fiberoptic bronchoscopy was also performed in the 32 asthmatics. The study was aimed at measuring FSTL1 levels. However, it was noted that IOS measurements in these patients were more sensitive than that of spirometry. FSTL1 levels were higher in asthmatics and improved with treatment. IOS showed more improvement than FEV1 in the same patients where the FSTL1 was decreased. Indirectly, therefore IOS may be considered a more accurate measurement of the inflammatory process and airway remodeling in the lung than spirometry [15].

8. IOS and beta-2 receptor polymorphism

Gly16Arg beta-2 receptor genotype is a variant allele in the polymorphism of Beta 2 adrenergic receptor family. In other words, in asthmatic children, the presence of this LDL is associated with sub-sensitivity response following exposure to regular long-acting beta-2 agonist in asthmatic patients receiving concurrent inhaled corticosteroids. In a study involving 112 patients treated with inhaled corticosteroids with a mean age of 43 years old, there was no difference in response to treatment with inhaled corticosteroids or combination of inhaled corticosteroids with long-acting beta agonist in terms of IOS response. In other words, allelic variation of the beta-2 adrenergic receptor did not influence the IOS outcomes [16].

9. IOS and observations in pre-asthma

In a recent study, 21 school children participated in a 6-minute walk with a measurement of spirometry and IOS before the 6-minute walk, post 6-minute walk, followed by 30-minute of rest, and an additional 6-minute walk, IOS, and spirometry. One hundred twenty-three children participated, but only 21 school children were able to perform the spirometric maneuvers according to preestablished inclusion criteria. Of the 21 children, 9 were able to perform the 6-minute walk with no changes in the IOS. Significant increase in R5 as well as R20 was noted in the rest of the children who participated. Spirometry did not change, but there was a decrease in the FEF 25–75%. The importance of this study is that it suggests that greater attention should be given to submaximal test particularly in children who are predisposed to airway alterations [17].

On the other hand, body mass index status can play an important role in the baseline reactance curve in children who are between the ages of 8 and 16 years. At the age of 16 years, there was increased blood neutrophil count in overweight obese girls but not in boys. However, both genders showed increased reactance or AX even though these patients were not complaining of symptoms to suggest asthma. The nitric oxide washout was normal in this population. The R5 was higher in this age group. IOS therefore can be a predictor of possible asthma in adolescence with high BMI [18].

Passive smoking may result in alteration of pulmonary function in infants born preterm. A study of 139 children between the ages of 3 and 7 years old who were born late preterm were categorized whether they had presence or absence of exposure to passive smoking. Patients who are exposed to passive smoking had a higher R5 and are 5/20 as well as a higher AX than patients who were not exposed to passive smoking. Passive smoking therefore can be a factor in early asthma development particularly in this patient population [19].

In conclusion, IOS or impulse oscillometry has been shown to reflect improvement in lung function following short-acting beta agonist treatment, as well as with long-term use of inhaled corticosteroids or combination of inhaled corticosteroids with long-acting beta agonist. The improvement was noted in multiple studies to be independent of the change or status of routine spirometry. It may also provide a better assessment of small airways through its R5 and AX measurements.

In addition, IOS can be more useful and effort independent in measurement of airway hyperresponsiveness in adults and children. It appears to be along with the measurement of nitric oxide exhalation to be reflective of the status of airway inflammation. The observed improvement and IOS are independent of the allele change or polymorphism of the beta-2 adrenergic receptor. It can play a role in the detection of early asthma particularly in children who are obese or exposed to passive smoking. This can be detected either by baseline IOS measurement or following 6-minute walk.

Monoclonal antibodies have been used in the treatment of severe asthma. These are patients who are either unresponsive to high-dose inhaled corticosteroids or are unable to be weaned off by oral corticosteroids. These patients have at least two exacerbations within 6 months. In following these patients, there is very limited data about the role of IOS at baseline and during follow-up. We have published data in an abstract form on 12 patients who were on omalizumab that showed improvement in the IOS but not spirometry with follow-up. These patients also improved in terms of tapering high-dose inhaled corticosteroids or oral steroids and had a decrease in their exacerbations even though there was no change in their FEV1. Future studies in this regard in patients with high IgE and eosinophilic asthma are warranted.

10. Role of IOS and COPD

In patients with COPD, it is well known that spirometry can be used to define the GOLD criteria. In other words, the FEV1 and the FVC are important parameters in defining the stage of the GOLD criteria. However, in general patients with COPD or chronic obstructive pulmonary disease had very little change upon follow-up in terms of improvement in the lung function based on the spirometry. Therefore, the most reliable current guidelines include quality of life, smoking cessation, 6-minute walk, oxygenation, and perhaps improvement in the FEV1. There have been several reports that showed that the impulse oscillometry can improve even though the spirometry does not change both in terms of short-term treatment with short-acting beta agonists and long-acting beta agonist/long-acting muscarinic antagonists with or without inhaled corticosteroids.

A study of 215 participants IOS was studied in the setting of chronic obstructive pulmonary disease or COPD of which 18, 83, 78, and 36 patients were classified under the GOLD criteria as grade 1, 2, 3, and 4, respectively. IOS parameters showed worsening of R5 and reactance or AX depending upon the severity of their COPD. There was a negative correlation with spirometry at baseline. This study recorded IOS at baseline, and it showed good correlation with traditional pulmonary parameters. The conclusion was that IOS can be used as an alternative methodology for evaluation of patients with COPD [1].

The diagnosis of COPD can be difficult at times particularly in the early stages. Thirty-five patients who had moderate to severe COPD showed improvement both in the AX and the resistance in the small airways following treatment with long-acting beta agonist/long-acting muscarinic antagonist combination. The improvement was more prominent than the improvement noted in the FEV1. In fact, FEV1 and FVC statistical significance for the small sample size was not present. IOS improvement was noted in follow-up visit of these patients [20].

Another study evaluated IOS in a pediatric patients, in the use of combination of fluticasone and salmeterol combined with tiotropium, there was significant improvement in R5 and AX in patients who received the triple combination as compared to patients who only received tiotropium by itself. In this study, spirometric findings were also noted to improve with the triple combination. However, IOS findings appear to be more significant. The conclusion by the authors is that IOS may provide a physiological point of view that is different from spirometry and seemed to be applicable as an additional assessment tool targeting COPD patients [21].

These patients were noted at baseline to improve in terms of IOS even though the spirometry did not change. There was also improvement in the impulse oscillometry or AX with follow-up. Statistical significance was noted with improvement in AX, R5, and R15 despite the lack of improvement in FEV1. In conclusion, there was improvement in the impulse oscillometry at baseline as well as maintenance follow-up therapy in patients with mild to moderate COPD.

Peripheral airway dysfunction was also noted in COPD patients who experience sleep disturbance. Fifty patients were evaluated in the morning after sleep. Questionnaires were given about the quality of sleep. IOS measurements were noted to be abnormal particularly increased AX and R5. The study demonstrated that sleep disturbances due to COPD symptoms are associated with airway constriction which is reflective of peripheral airway dysfunction [22].

On the whole, the studies suggest that impulse oscillometry may offer a new clue in the diagnosis and follow-up of patients with COPD. The limitation of the studies is that a combination of asthma and COPD cannot be entirely excluded. It has been suggested that nitric oxide measurement is helpful in the differentiation of combination of asthma/COPD and COPD. In patients with COPD by itself, nitric oxide measurement in the exhaled breath is usually very low and is in general less than 5. However, further studies in this regard are needed to reaffirm these findings.

11. IOS and other respiratory conditions

Cystic fibrosis is a multisystem disease with respiratory system involvement responsible for 90% of morbidity and mortality. Conventional spirometry is considered the main method to evaluate airway disease in patients with cystic fibrosis. FEV1 has been recognized as an objective parameter to evaluate the course of the disease and response to treatment. Forty-nine cystic fibrosis patients between the ages 3 and 18 were compared to 45 healthy controls. IOS was performed in both groups. Spirometry was also performed in patients who are more than 6 years old, while patients who were less than 6 years old only had IOS. In both groups, it was noted that the resistance increased and so did the AX during exacerbation and decreased after treatment. This was independent of the bronchodilator effects. IOS therefore may be useful to evaluate pulmonary function and detect acute exacerbation in cystic fibrosis patients [23].

Hypersensitivity pneumonitis is a complex clinical syndrome that results from abnormal immune lung function to diverse inhaled antigens. It can be related to protein antigens denied from birds as well as air conditioning and can progress to pulmonary fibrosis. Small airway involvement is associated with interstitial mononuclear infiltrate with non-necrotizing poorly formed granulomas and varying degree of fibrosis. Therefore, detection of small airway dysfunction is essential in establishing the severity of the disease process. In a study of 20 consecutive patients with established diagnosis of hypersensitivity pneumonitis, there was ventilation perfusion mismatch. IOS was obtained, and it did show elevated AX at baseline and improved with treatment particularly with azathioprine and prednisone. It is noted that lung volume also improved but not gas exchange [24].

A case report in 2005 demonstrated a lung transplant patient who had deterioration in the IOS even though the spirometry did not change. The AX was worse and so was the resistance in the small and large airways. This was reflective of early transplant rejection. The usefulness of IOS in monitoring lung transplant patient was evaluated by Dr. Ochman and published in 2018. The study involved 25 consecutive patients with successful lung transplantation, and 88% of these patients were noted to have increased AX indicating peripheral airway obstruction. There was an increase in the small airway resistance or R5 as well. The median age was 46 years old. This was a baseline study but suggested that IOS measurements may also be important in evaluating possible early rejection in patients with lung transplant [25].

Finally, it is well noted that vocal cord disorder in patients with chronic cough, uncontrolled COPD, or severe asthma can be a contributing factor to the worsening of the symptoms. We have noted that a ratio of AX on inspiration/AX expiration of greater than 2 is consistent with vocal cord disorder. Improvement in vocal cord disorder such as treatment of asymptomatic reflux, increased postnasal drip, and vocal cord dysfunction can lead to secondary improvement in asthma and other related conditions.

12. Conclusion

The clinical utility of IOS in asthma is well established. IOS is a noninvasive tool that is independent of patient effort and reproducible in pediatric and adult patients. IOS serves as a technique that can be used with spirometry or independently to diagnose and manage asthma. In addition, the utility of IOS is expanding and has shown to be useful in COPD and other inflammatory lung diseases.

Author details

Constantine Saadeh[1,2,3]* and Nicole Davey-Ranasinghe[1,2,3]

1 Amarillo Center for Clinical Research (ACCR), Texas, USA

2 Allergy, Asthma, Rheumatology Treatment Specialists (Allergy ARTS), Amarillo, Texas, USA

3 Texas Tech University Health Sciences Center, Texas, USA

*Address all correspondence to: aarts@allergyarts.com

References

[1] Wei X, Shi Z, Cui Y, Mi J, Ma Z, Ren J, et al. Impulse oscillometry system as an alternative diagnostic method for chronic obstructive pulmonary disease. Medicine. 2017;**96**(46):e8543

[2] Saadeh C et al. Retrospective observation on the ability to diagnose and manage patients with asthma through the use of impulse oscillometry: Comparison with spirometry and overview of the literature. Pulmonary Medicine. 2014;**2014**:376890. 9 pages

[3] Kjellberg S, Houltz BK, Zetterstrom O, Robinson PD, Gustafsson PM. Clinical characteristics of adult asthma associated with small airway dysfunction. Respiratory Medicine. 2016;**117**:92-102

[4] Kalliola S, Malmberg LP, Pelkonen AS, Mäkelä MJ. Aberrant small airways function relates to asthma severity in young children. Respiratory Medicine. 2016;**111**:16-20. DOI: 10.1016/j.rmed.2015.12.006

[5] Galant SP, Komarow HD, Shin HW, Siddiqui S, Lipworth BJ. The case for impulse oscillometry in the management of asthma in children and adults. Annals of Allergy, Asthma & Immunology. 2017;**118**(6):664-671. DOI: 10.1016/j.anai.2017.04.009

[6] Boudewijn IM, Postma DS, Telenga ED, Ten Hacken NH, Timens W, Oudkerk M, et al. Effects of ageing and smoking on pulmonary computed tomography scans using parametric response mapping. The European Respiratory Journal. 2015;**46**(4):1193-1196. DOI: 10.1183/09031936.00009415

[7] Carr TF, Altisheh R, Zitt M. Small airways disease and severe asthma. World Allergy Organization Journal. 2017;**10**(1):20. DOI: 10.1186/s40413-017-0153-4

[8] van Veen IH, Ten Brinke A, Sterk PJ, Sont JK, Gauw SA, Rabe KF, et al. Exhaled nitric oxide predicts lung function decline in difficult-to-treat asthma. The European Respiratory Journal. 2008;**32**(2):344-349. DOI: 10.1183/09031936.00135907

[9] Mansura AH, Manneya S, Ayresb JG. Methacholine-induced asthma symptoms correlate with impulse oscillometry but not spirometry. Respiratory Medicine. 2008;**102**:42-49

[10] Cox CA, Boudewijn IM, Vroegop SJ, Schokker S, Lexmond AJ, Frijlink HW, et al. Associations of AMP and adenosine induced dyspnea sensation to large and small airways dysfunction in asthma. BMC Pulmonary Medicine. 2019;**19**(1):23. DOI: 10.1186/s12890-019-0783-0

[11] Lajunen K, Kalliola S, Kotaniemi-Syrjänen A, Sarna S, Malmberg LP, Pelkonen AS, et al. Abnormal lung function at preschool age asthma in adolescence. Annals of Allergy, Asthma & Immunology. 2018;**120**(5):520-526. DOI: 10.1016/j.anai.2018.03.002

[12] Schulze J, Biedebach S, Christmann M, Herrmann E, Voss S, Zielen S. Impulse oscillometry as a predictor of asthma exacerbations in young children. Respiration. 2016;**91**(2):107-114. DOI: 10.1159/000442448

[13] Short PM, Anderson WJ, Manoharan A, Lipworth BJ. Usefulness of impulse oscillometry for the assessment of airway hyperresponsiveness in mild-to-moderate adult asthma. Annals of Allergy, Asthma & Immunology. 2015;**115**(1):17-20. DOI: 10.1016/j.anai.2015.04.022

[14] Wasilewski VN, Fisher T, Turcotte SE, Fisher JT, Lougheed MD. Bronchodilating effect of deep

inspirations in asthma and chronic cough. Journal of Applied Physiology. 2016;**120**(9):1018-1028. DOI: 10.1152/japplphysiol.00737.2015

[15] Liu Y, Liu T, Wu J, Li T, Jiao X, Zhang H, et al. The correlation between FSTL1 expression and airway remodeling in asthmatics. Mediators of Inflammation. 2017;**2017**:7918472. DOI: 10.1155/2017/7918472

[16] Jabbal S, Manoharan A, Lipworth J, Anderson W, Short P, Lipworth B. Is Gly16Arg β2 receptor polymorphism related to impulse oscillometry in a real-life asthma clinic setting. Lung. 2016;**194**(2):267-271. DOI: 10.1007/s00408-016-9848-5

[17] Assumpção MS, Ribeiro JD, Wamosy RMG, Parazzi PLF, Schivinski CIS. Impulse oscillometry and spirometry in schoolers submitted to the six-minute walk test. Revista Paulista de Pediatria. 2018;**36**(4):474-481. DOI: 10.1590/1984-0462/;2018;36;4;00007

[18] Ekström S, Hallberg J, Kull I, Protudjer JLP, Thunqvist P, Bottai M, et al. Body mass index status and peripheral airway obstruction in school-age children: A population-based cohort study. Thorax. 2018;**73**(6):538-545. DOI: 10.1136/thoraxjnl-2017-210716

[19] Gunlemez A, Er İ, Baydemir C, Arisoy A. Effects of passive smoking on lung function tests in preschool children born late-preterm: A preventable health priority. The Journal of Maternal-Fetal & Neonatal Medicine. 2018;**1**:1-6. DOI: 10.1080/14767058.2018.1430759

[20] Molino A, Simioli F, Stanziola AA, Mormile M, Martino M, D'Amato M. Effects of combination therapy indacaterol/glycopyrronium versus tiotropium on moderate to severe COPD: Evaluation of impulse oscillometry and exacerbation rate. Multidisciplinary Respiratory Medicine. 2017;**12**:25. DOI: 10.1186/s40248-017-0105-4

[21] Mineshita M, Shikama Y, Nakajima H, Nishihira R, Komatsu S, Kubota M, et al. The application of impulse oscillation system for the evaluation of treatment effects in patients with COPD. Respiratory Physiology & Neurobiology. 2014;**202**: 1-5. DOI: 10.1016/j.resp.2014.07.008

[22] Basile M, Baiamonte P, Mazzuca E, Principe S, Pennavaria F, Benfante A, et al. Sleep disturbances in COPD are associated with heterogeneity of airway obstruction. COPD. 2018;**15**(4):350-354. DOI: 10.1080/15412555.2018.1504015

[23] Sakarya A, Uyan ZS, Baydemir C, Anık Y, Erdem E, Gokdemir Y, et al. Evaluation of children with cystic fibrosis by impulse oscillometry when stable and at exacerbation. Pediatric Pulmonology. 2016;**51**(11):1151-1158. DOI: 10.1002/ppul.23449

[24] Guerrero Zúñiga S, Sánchez Hernández J, Mateos Toledo H, Mejía Ávila M, Gochicoa-Rangel L, Miguel Reyes JL, et al. Small airway dysfunction in chronic hypersensitivity pneumonitis. Respirology. 2017;**22**(8):1637-1642. DOI: 10.1111/resp.13124

[25] Ochman M, Wojarski J, Wiórek A, Slezak W, Maruszewski M, Karolak W, et al. Usefulness of the impulse oscillometry system in graft function monitoring in lung transplant recipients. Transplantation Proceedings. 2018;**50**(7):2070-2074. DOI: 10.1016/j.transproceed.2017.12.060

[26] Saadeh C, Saadeh C, Cross B, Gaylor M, Griffith M. Advantage of impulse oscillometry over spirometry to diagnose chronic obstructive pulmonary disease and monitor pulmonary responses to bronchodilators: An observational study. SAGE Open Medicine. 2015;**3**:2050312115578957. DOI: 10.1177/2050312115578957

[27] Sol IS, Kim YH, Kim S, Kim JD, Choi SH, Kim KW, et al. Assessment of withinbreath impulse oscillometry parameters in children with asthma. Pediatric Pulmonology. 2019;**54**(2): 117-124. DOI:10.1002/ppul.24201

[28] Zeng J, Chen Z, Hu Y, Hu Q, Zhong S, Liao W. Asthma control in preschool children with small airway function as measured by IOS and fractional exhaled nitric oxide. Respiratory Medicine. 2018;**145**:8-13. DOI: 10.1016/j.rmed.2018.10.009

Chapter 3

Role of Airway Smooth Muscle Cells in Asthma Pathology

Wenchao Tang

Abstract

Airway smooth muscle (ASM) cells have been shown to play an important role in bronchial asthma. As the research progresses, the mechanism becomes more and more complex. This chapter reviews the role of ASM in asthma pathological mechanisms including inflammatory reaction, extracellular matrix proteins, cell contraction, cell structure, neuromodulation, airway remodeling, apoptosis, autophagy, miRNA, mitochondria, etc. In brief, ASM is similar to a "processing station." It is not only affected by various signals in the body to produce biological effects and secrete various signals to act on downstream target cells but also feeds back to the upstream pathways or receives feedback from downstream pathways to form a complex network. The results summarized in this chapter are expected to provide new targets for the clinical treatment of asthma.

Keywords: airway smooth muscle cells, asthma, inflammation, airway hyperreactivity, airway remodeling

1. Introduction

Bronchial asthma is a chronic airway inflammatory disease involving a variety of airway inflammatory cells, airway structural cells, and cellular components of which airway smooth muscle (ASM) cells have received the most intensive investigation. ASM has been shown to play an important role in the structure, function, and contraction of the airways. Evidence suggests that some ASM signaling mechanisms can help regulate the release of pro-inflammatory and anti-inflammatory mediators, which are factors that regulate immunity; different types of airway cells (such as epithelial cells, fibroblasts, and nerve cells); intracellular Ca^{2+} concentration-mediated airway contraction and relaxation; cell proliferation and apoptosis, autophagy, production, and regulation of the extracellular matrix (ECM); and neuromodulation. These mechanisms cause structural changes in the narrowing and dilatation of the airway, resulting in airway hyperreactivity (AHR) and airway stenosis, hence affecting airway compliance.

2. ASM participates in asthma by releasing pro-inflammatory or anti-inflammatory factors and immune regulators

ASM can produce a variety of pro-inflammatory and anti-inflammatory factors triggered by inflammation, injuries, and microbial products [1], including interleukin-1β (IL-1β), IL-5, IL-6, IL-8, IL-17, platelet-derived growth factor

(PDGF), transforming growth factor-β (TGF-β), etc., which constitute a complex network that participates in airway inflammation. For example, IL-6 induces ASM cell proliferation and further modulates immune cell function [2], and TNF-α exerts its mediating effects by enhancing interferon (IFNβ) secretion [3]. Recent studies have confirmed that ASM can produce and release thymic stromal lymphopoietin (TSLP) and can also act as a target of TSLP to participate in the recruitment of dendritic cells to regulate airway immune responses [4, 5]. ASM cells also produce chemokines such as RANTES and eotaxin [6]. The specific mechanism may be mediated by mitogen-activated protein kinase (MAPK), janus kinase/signal transducer and activator of transcription protein signaling pathway (JAK/Stat), and c-jun N-terminal kinase (JNK) [7, 8]. There is also evidence that ASM can also secrete growth factors such as vascular endothelial growth factor (VEGF) and brain-derived neurotrophic factor (BNDF), and these growth factors may be involved in ASM proliferation and contraction through autocrine effects [9].

3. ASM acts on asthma by secreting extracellular matrix (ECM)

The action of ASM ECM proteins on airway remodeling by autocrine or paracrine effects is a current research focus in asthma. ASM can produce a series of ECM proteins [10]. In the airway, ECM proteins surround cells in the form of reticular collagen or noncollagen, and their density and structure affect cellular characteristics such as proliferation, migration, differentiation, and survival. The related components include collagen, fibronectin, the matrix metalloprotein (MMP) family (MMP-2, MMP-3, MMP-9, MMP-13, etc.), and metalloprotein antagonists (TIMP-1 and TIMP-2) (**Figure 1**) [1, 11, 12]. Meanwhile, ECM protein signaling groups can in turn regulate other cells such as epithelial cells and ASMs. The ECM can control its own conformation, release growth factors, and MMPs and regulate the activity of local growth factors (such as neurotrophin and VEGF) and cytokines by cleavage

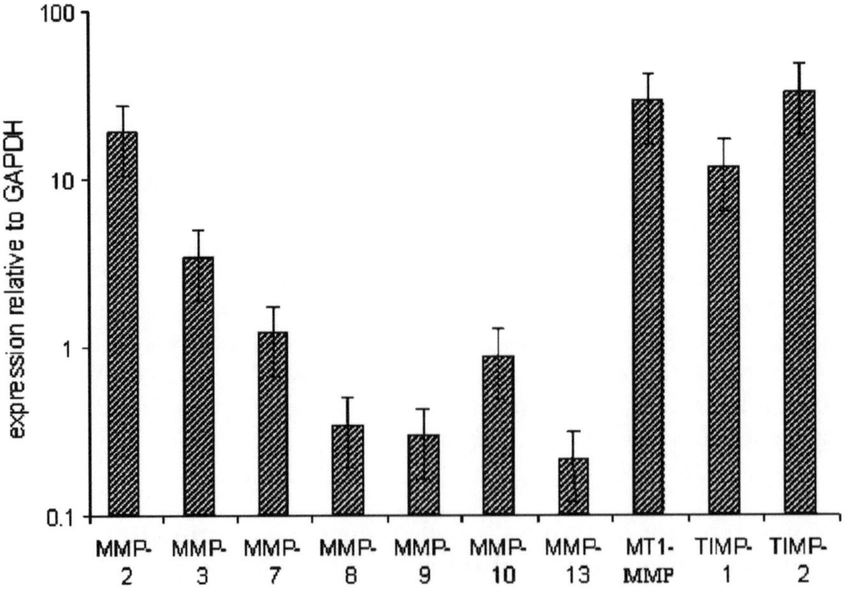

Figure 1.
MMP and TIMP mRNA expression by qRT-PCR five primary ASM cell cultures and expressed relative to GAPDH. It was originally published on "Matrix metalloproteinase expression and activity in human airway smooth muscle cells" of the British Journal of Pharmacology by Shona R. Elshaw et al.

and inactivation [13], thereby forming a complex signaling network to regulate airway remodeling. For example, IL-1β can interact with tumor necrosis factor-α (TNF-α), thus increasing MMP-12 [14] and MMP-9 [15], promoting cell migration and remodeling, and further regulating growth factor activity.

In terms of the regulatory mechanisms of the ECM, Rho kinase inhibitors can prevent ECM-induced airway remodeling [16]. The Wnt/β-catenin pathway can regulate TGF-β regulation of ASM-derived ECM [1, 17]. In contrast, decorin (an ECM proteoglycan) binds to TGF-β and reduces ECM production [18]. Even infections can regulate ECM products via ASM, and rhinovirus-induced infections increase fibronectin and basement membrane glycans, especially in the ASM of asthma patients [19]. Thus, altering the production of ECM, thereby modulating the inflammatory mediators or growth factors produced by the ASM or other cells, may result in cross reaction of airway structures and functions.

4. ASM is involved in asthma through other mechanisms

In addition to inflammatory mediators and growth factors, many emerging mechanisms have been reported to be involved in ASM and airway remodeling. For example, vitamin D has been shown to inhibit remodeling in vitro and in vivo [20]. However, its mechanism involving airway ASM cells is still under investigation [21]. Another emerging mechanism is thyroxine, which has been reported to enhance ASM proliferation [22], while low thyroxine levels cause airway developmental malformations [23]. Some reports also suggest that insulin appears to enhance ASM proliferation and ECM formation [24]. In addition, sphingolipids participate in airway inflammation, AHR, and remodeling. In particular, sphingosine-1-phosphate can promote ASM contractility and regulate inflammation and airway remodeling [25, 26].

5. Roles of ASM, $[Ca^{2+}]_i$, and contraction mechanisms in asthma

The cytosolic Ca^{2+} concentration ($[Ca^{2+}]_i$) is a well-established pathway for the regulation of ASM contraction. The $[Ca^{2+}]_i$ can affect voltage-gated channels, receptor-regulated channels, and calcium pool-regulated channels. These channels are subjected to regulation by pathways such as phospholipase C (PLC), inositol triphosphate (IP3), ryanodine receptor (RyR), etc. (**Figure 2**). Meanwhile, sarco/endoplasmic reticulum Ca^{2+} ATPase (SERCA), bidirectional Na^{+}-Ca^{2+} exchangers (NCX), and mitochondrial buffers can limit $[Ca^{2+}]_i$ and regulate calcium storage by inhibiting the activation of $[Ca^{2+}]_i$. In addition to $[Ca^{2+}]_i$, Ca^{2+}-calmodulin-dependent myosin light chain (MLC) kinase and MLC act in tandem to regulate ASM contractility by excitatory myosin interaction. Studies have shown that the Rho-associated coiled-coil containing kinases (ROCK) pathway inhibits the contraction of Ca^{2+}-sensitive cells by inhibiting the sensitivity of MLC kinase [27]. IP3 can activate Ca^{2+} influx [28] in ASM and regulate local Ca^{2+} release [29].

5.1 GPCR mechanism and asthma

G-protein-coupled receptors (GPCRs) are a superfamily of cell membrane proteins that transduce extracellular signals, causing intracellular cascades and leading to different cellular functions. This mechanism is used to treat diseases such as asthma and chronic obstructive pulmonary disease (COPD). In ASM, most of the existing research focuses on the expression and function of different GPCRs (G_q, G_i, and G_s) in ASM contraction/relaxation. For instance, traditional

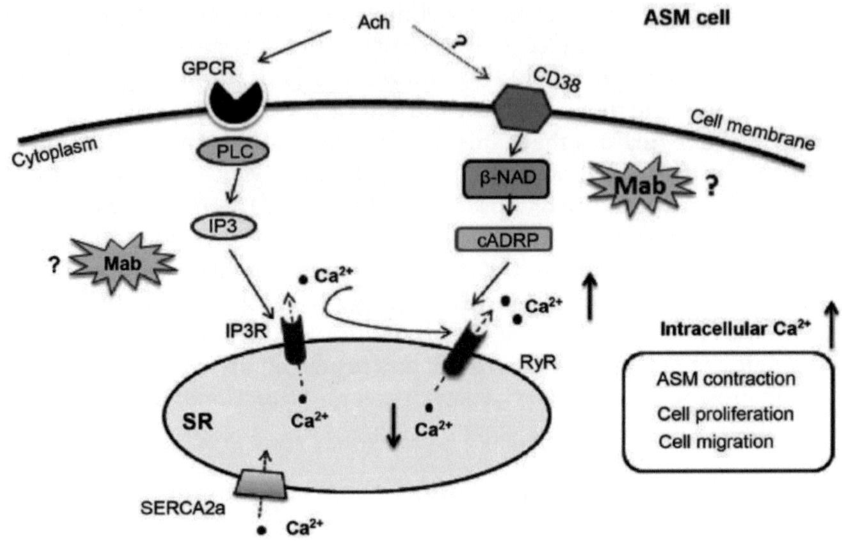

Figure 2.
Signaling pathways of Ca^{2+} concentration in ASM involving IP3R and RyR and the potential targets of mabuterol hydrochloride (Mab) that intervene in the increased level of intracellular Ca^{2+} induced with Ach. Binding with a G-protein-coupled receptor, Ach activates PLC to generate IP3, which encourages the clusters of IP3R on SR to release Ca^{2+}. RyR may also be activated or potentiated by cADP ribose (cADPR). It may be sequestered by the superficial sarcoplasmic reticulum (SR) through sarcoendoplasmic Ca^{2+} ATPase 2a (SERCA2a), although much of the calcium is released from stores and enters the cytoplasm. The increased level of intracellular Ca^{2+} leads to the contraction, proliferation, and migration of the ASM. It was originally published on "Matrix metalloproteinase expression and activity in human airway smooth muscle cells" of the British Journal of Pharmacology by Shona R. Elshaw et al. It was originally published on "Suppression of the increasing level of acetylcholine-stimulated intracellular Ca2+ in guinea pig airway smooth muscle cells by mabuterol" of Biomedical Reports by Xirui Song et al.

bronchoconstrictor agonists such as acetylcholine (ACh), histamine, and endothelin act through the G_q-coupled pathway, activating the PLC-IP3 pathway and thereby increasing Ca^{2+}. However, bronchiectasis caused by the G_s-coupled pathway (increasing cAMP) is the major mechanism of action of the β2-adrenergic receptor [30]. Moreover, GPCRs alone or in combination with other pathways, such as receptor tyrosine kinases acting through cell proliferation/growth, secretion of growth factors, and inflammatory mediators, promote the "synthesis function" of ASM, and its remodeling of airways is gaining increasing attention [31].

The current common GPCRs include gamma-aminobutyric acid (GABA), calcium-sensing receptor (CaSR), thromboxane (TXA2), bitter taste receptor (BTR), and prostaglandin E2 (PGE2). The present research status is summarized as follows.

GABA is a major inhibitory neurotransmitter in the mammalian central nervous system and activates both the ligand-gated ionotropic GABAA receptor and the G-protein-coupled metabotropic GABAB receptor. Functional GABAB receptors are present in ASM [32, 33] and airway epithelium [34]. GABAB produces airway contraction through G_i, and the GABAA receptor on ASM appears to be a potent bronchodilator [35]. Since the human ASM GABAA receptor only expresses the α4 and α5 subunits, recent studies have shown that selective targeting of the ASM GABAA receptor can improve the efficacy of anti-asthmatic drugs and minimize side effects [36]. The reported data suggest that the heterogeneity of selective targeting of ASM GABAA receptor features is a novel approach to bronchiectasis.

CaSR, a GPCR, is often expressed in non-Ca^{2+}-regulated tissues such as blood vessels and breasts and can regulate the extracellular Ca^{2+} concentration ($[Ca^{2+}]_e$), gene expression, ion channels, and ECM through the parathyroid glands, kidneys, and bones. Abnormal expression of CaSR is usually associated with inflammation, vascular calcification, and tumors. Although CaSR is important in the development of the lungs, studies on the expression or function of CaSR in the airways are still rare. CaSR has been reported to be expressed in the developing airway epithelium [37] and regulates the morphology of the lung bronchus through $[Ca^{2+}]_e$ levels, thereby affecting tracheal remodeling [38]. In adults, CaSR is present in the human respiratory tract, especially in ASM, and CaSR expression is increased in ASM of asthmatic subjects [39], which may become a new target for future asthma treatment. Depending on the cell type, the expression and function of CaSR are regulated by signaling pathways such as ROCK, extracellular signal-regulated kinase (ERKs), and protein kinase C (PKC) [40]. Therefore, this receptor can be considered a multimode sensor and effector for the integration of composite signals and has an important impact on airway structure and function.

TXA2 is a potent endogenous bronchoconstrictor that is observed to have increased levels in asthmatic airways [41]. TXA2 induces and enhances the contraction of allergic bronchi primarily through interaction with the thromboxane prostaglandin (TP) receptor coupled to G_q and the PLC/IP3/Ca^{2+} pathway. Studies have shown that the TXA2 effector mechanism is complex and involves indirect effects of neuronal stimulation leading to ACh release and mechanical stimulation [42].

The BTR is a recently discovered bronchodilator. It was originally thought to act through the taste 2 receptors (TAS2R) family of GPCRs to increase $[Ca^{2+}]_i$ and induce bronchiectasis [43]. TAS2Rs exhibit low specificity and affinity for a wide range of bitter compounds, and the corresponding result is a diversity of signal combinations. Factors affecting TAS2Rs include agonist concentration and receptor desensitization [44]. BTR can induce membrane hyperpolarization [45] via the blocker-sensitive Ca^{2+}-activated K-channels [43, 46] and nonselective cation channels and interact with specific bronchoconstrictors [46]. Moreover, studies have suggested that BTRs can activate different Ca^{2+} signaling pathways under specific conditions. For example, TAS2R stimulation activates Gβγ under baseline conditions to increase $[Ca^{2+}]_i$ [47]. Other studies have also shown that the bronchodilating effect of BTR may also depend on interactions with β2-adrenergic receptor expression and signaling [48]. When TAS2R is activated, relaxation can be induced even under adrenergic receptor desensitization [48], which may be an alternative treatment method for asthma patients with bronchiectasis who are desensitized to β-agonists. Through extensive research, BTR has also been shown to affect genetic variations that result in sinusitis and asthma [49]; the mechanism by which BTR relaxes the airway has not yet been elucidated.

PGE2 and its epoprostenol (EP) receptor subtype are produced by airway epithelium and ASM and have complex effects on bronchoconstriction and expansion. Previous studies have shown that endogenous PGE2 has a bronchial protective effect in asthma. The PGE2 signal acts through four different GPCRs (EP1–EP4). Since different pathways have different G-protein coupling and downstream signals, and some downstream pathways can counteract each other [50], the mechanism of action is complicated. Studies have shown that EP1 increases Ca^{2+} and EP3 reduces cAMP synthesis, leading to ASM contraction, while EP2 and EP4 induce bronchodilation by increasing cAMP. In addition, EP3 can also cause an opposite reaction by promoting ASM migration [51].

In addition to the above GPCR-related mechanisms, many studies have been performed on Wnt signaling in the airways in recent years. Wnt proteins act through coreceptors such as lipoprotein receptor-associated protein (LRP)-5/LRP-6, receptor-like tyrosine kinase (Ryk), and receptor tyrosine kinase-like orphan receptor 2 (Ror2) to promote binding to the extracellular domain of the frizzled (Frz) family of GPCRs. The Wnt signaling pathways include the classical β-catenin-dependent and β-catenin-independent pathways and the noncanonical Wnt/Ca^{2+} pathway. In ASM, Wnt signaling is thought to be closely related to airway remodeling [52].

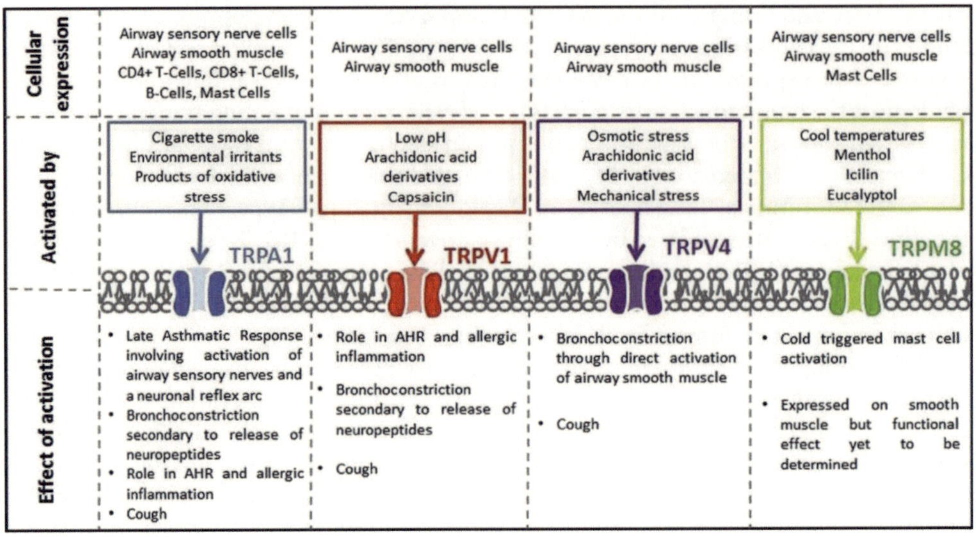

Figure 3.
The role of TRP channels in ASM. It was originally published on "Novel drug targets for asthma and COPD: Lessons learned from in vitro and in vivo models" of Pulmonary Pharmacology & Therapeutics by Katie E. Baker et al.

In fibroblasts, Wnt5B can increase the secretion of IL-6 and chemokine ligand 8 (CXCL-8) and indirectly affect airway remodeling (69). In epithelial cells, Wnt signaling in inflammation produces ECM and indirectly induces remodeling [53].

5.2 Non-GPCR mechanisms and asthma

Regarding airway contraction controlled by non-GPCR mechanisms, the mechanism of Ca^{2+} signaling regulation has been intensely investigated. For example, calcineurin can regulate local Ca^{2+} signaling and contractility in ASM. Meanwhile, the Ca^{2+} influx channel TRPC3 can activate the calcineurin/nuclear factor of activated T cells (NFAT) pathway to regulate airway contraction [54].

In addition, ASM can also express some specific receptors such as the transient receptor potential ankyrin 1 (TRPA1) or polysaccharides for non-GPCR-mediated airway regulation. In particular, TRPA1 and capsaicin receptor 1 (TRPV1) channels can be activated by PKC resulting in neuromodulation of airway contraction [55]. Studies have shown that ASM expresses TRPA1 [56] and TRPV1 [57] as well as TRPV4 [58, 59]. TRPA1 has been shown to promote IL-8 secretion in ASM, enhance airway inflammation and AHR [60], and mobilize $[Ca^{2+}]_i$ [56] while inhibiting the proliferation of ASM [61]. In contrast, TRPV1 appears to promote proliferation [62]. TRPV4 is associated with an increase in $[Ca^{2+}]_i$ [59] and ASM contraction and proliferation (**Figure 3**) [58, 63]. In addition to TRPA, ASM can also express epidermal growth factor receptor (EGFR) and hyaluronic acid to participate in airway inflammation [64]. The expression of hyaluronic acid is increased during inflammation [65] and is involved in the homeostasis of aqueous fluids, cell matrix signaling, cell proliferation and migration, and regulation of inflammation [66].

6. ASM cell structure and asthma

Some intracellular and extracellular structures of ASM are closely related to the pathological changes of asthma. Caveolae and their regulatory caveolin and cavin proteins are a focus of research. Caveolae have been shown to contain excitatory contractile receptors and activate Ca^{2+} influx channels (including transient receptor potential channel (TRPC) subtypes and calcium release-activated calcium channel protein 1 (Orai1)) [67, 68]. The decreased expression of its important component, caveolin-1, induces an increase in ASM $[Ca^{2+}]_i$ and a contractile response and promotes ASM proliferation [69]. The relevant mechanisms include a reduction in $[Ca^{2+}]_i$ influx, increase in sarcoplasmic reticulum Ca^{2+} release, and reduction in Ca^{2+} sensitivity through the RhoA pathway. Conversely, pro-inflammatory factors such as TNF-α can enhance the expression and function of caveolin-1 [70].

7. Proliferation and apoptosis of ASM cells and airway remodeling during asthma

Airway remodeling is an important pathological change in asthma. The increased mass of ASM may be a key feature of airway remodeling, and its hyperplasia and hypertrophy are unevenly distributed in bronchi of different sizes. This process can enhance airway contraction and airway stenosis, further leading to decreased lung function or severe asthma [71]. The underlying causes of ASM hypertrophy have been extensively explored. For example, excessive mechanical stretching can lead to the release of EGF, which participates in remodeling [72]. In addition, Wnt, glycogen synthase kinase 3 beta (GSK3β) [73], or rapamycin target protein (mTOR) [74] may also be involved in the regulation of reconfiguration caused by mechanical forces. Studies have also shown that hypertrophy is associated with increased MLC kinase in ASM [75]. In addition, many signaling pathways have been found to be related to ASM proliferation, including p38, p42/p44 MAP kinase and PI3/Akt.

During the pathogenesis of asthma, some pro-inflammatory mediators are involved in the regulation of ASM proliferation, such as TNF-α, IL-4, IL-5, IL-13, TGF-β, thymic stromal lymphopoietin (TSLP), and Th17 family members. In addition, some conventional stimuli such as agonists of airway bronchial contraction [76] and other locally produced factors [9, 77] may also trigger an increase in proliferation under certain circumstances. Recent studies have shown that a nonreceptor tyrosine kinase, Abl, promotes ASM mitosis and enhances ASM proliferation [78]. It has also been suggested that sex hormones can affect the structure and function of the airway because, in some cases, estrogen can reduce mitosis and exert antiproliferative effects in the airway [79]. In addition, within ASM cells, microRNAs are thought to play an important role in the regulation of ASM cell proliferation and migration [80].

Overall, current information indicates that the interaction of multiple signaling mechanisms leads to airway remodeling represented by ASM cell proliferation. Although many inflammatory pathways can cause cell proliferation, limited data exist regarding how to inhibit or block proliferation. Studies have shown that regulating the ECM (such as the collagen density) or inducing increased expression of caveolin-1 can limit ASM cell proliferation [81] and some therapeutic drugs such as corticosteroids and β2 receptor agonists can also reduce proliferation [82]. In addition, peroxisome proliferator-activated receptor (PPAR)-γ ligands can attenuate ASM proliferation [83].

In the context of airway remodeling, an increase in ASM mass indicates an increase in cell proliferation and reflects a decrease in apoptosis. However, based on the current data, the mechanisms of the two are quite different. Th17-associated cytokines, IL-18, eotaxin, monocyte inflammatory protein-1a [84], and TRPV1 agonists [85] can alleviate ASM apoptosis. Other studies have found that peroxisome proliferator-activated receptor gamma (PPAR-γ) [86], collagen [87], and vitamin D can regulate ASM proliferation without affecting apoptosis.

8. ASM autophagy and asthma

At present, autophagy is considered an adaptive response of cells to survival that can promote cell death in the context of disease. This process is essential in maintaining homeostasis, managing external stress, and regulating cellular capacity. Autophagy plays a major role in the immune response to various pathogens, particularly viruses. In the case of asthma, autophagy in the airway epithelium or ASM may occur in the context of infection [88]. The current research on the role of autophagy in asthma and the types of cells involved is relatively limited. For example, pharmacological inhibition of gamma-glutamyltransferase 1 (GGT1) has been found to induce p53-dependent autophagy in human ASM cells [85]. In addition, excessive reactive oxygen species (ROS) that may be present during airway inflammation can induce autophagy, thus contributing to the pathophysiology of asthma [89].

9. ASM, miRNA, and asthma

Many studies have examined miRNA-mediated regulation of ASM. During the asthma process, many specific miRNAs are thought to play multiple roles in ASM [90]. For example, pro-inflammatory cytokines such as IL-1β, TNF-α, and IFNγ can downregulate 11 miRNAs, particularly miR-25, miR-140, miR-188, and miR-25. In contrast to the above results, another study [80] showed that expression levels of miR-146a and miR-146b were elevated in ASM in an IL-1β, TNF-α, and IFNγ-treated asthma group. Other studies have shown that only miR-146a is an endogenous negative regulator of human ASM cells [91].

In terms of airway remodeling, miR-140-3p regulates the important enzyme CD38 [92], which may have multiple downstream effects, such as affecting $[Ca^{2+}]_i$ and proliferation [93–95]. Under the induction of mechanical elongation, miR-26a causes ASM hypertrophy by attenuating GSK3β [96]. However, ASM proliferation appears to be driven by multiple miRNAs, including miR-10a [97], miR-23b [98], miR-138 [99], miR-145 [100], and miR-203 [101]. In general, we have found many miRNA pathways in ASM, but many problems remain unresolved, and miRNAs will be a focus for targeted asthma therapy in the future.

10. Mitochondria and ASM

Mitochondria in the airway not only produce ATP but are also involved in functions such as Ca^{2+} buffering [102–104], endoplasmic reticulum pathways, Ca^{2+} influx (such as store-operated Ca^{2+} entry (SOCE)), and cell proliferation and survival. These functions mostly involve fission and fusion of mitochondrial structures, mitochondrial biogenesis, mitochondrial autophagy, and ROS destruction [102, 105]. For example, consumption of mitochondrial DNA attenuates the concentration of $[Ca^{2+}]_i$ in ASM [106]. In terms of regulation, TGF-β enhances ASM mitochondrial ROS and promotes cytokine secretion [107]. Conversely, airway inflammation impairs mitochondrial Ca^{2+} buffering, resulting in an increase in $[Ca^{2+}]_i$. This damage leads to not only an increase in ROS but also an increase in endoplasmic reticulum stress and the unfolded protein response (UPR) [108]. These pathways are relevant because they can further influence protein expression and function as well as airway remodeling [109, 110].

11. Conclusions

With the rapid progress in molecular biology, cell biology, and various experimental techniques, research on ASM has developed rapidly, and an increasing number of functions have been discovered. When investigating ASM, we should consider the presence of surrounding cells and the ECM. Investigation of the role of ASM is no longer limited to its contractility, remodeling, and secretion. ASM is similar to a "processing station." It not only is affected by various signals in the body to produce biological effects and secrete various signals to act on downstream target cells but also feeds back to the upstream pathways or receives feedback from downstream pathways to form a complex network. Therefore, a univariant study of the mechanism of ASM action is unrealistic. More comprehensive studies integrating bioimaging, informatics, and other technologies are needed to conduct more accurate target interventions, obtain more precise pathway information, and provide new therapeutic targets for asthma.

Acknowledgements

This work was funded by the National Natural Science Foundation of China (grant number No. 81403469) and the Three-Year Development Plan Project for Traditional Chinese Medicine of Shanghai (grant number No. ZY (2018–2020)-CCCX-2001-2005).

Conflict of interest

The authors declare that they have no conflict of interest.

Author details

Wenchao Tang
School of Acupuncture-Moxibustion and Tuina, Shanghai University of Traditional Chinese Medicine, Shanghai, China

*Address all correspondence to: vincent.tang@shutcm.edu.cn

References

[1] Koziol-White CJ, Panettieri RA Jr. Airway smooth muscle and immunomodulation in acute exacerbations of airway disease. Immunological Reviews. 2011;**242**(1):178-185

[2] Robinson MB, Deshpande DA, Chou J, Cui W, Smith S, Langefeld C, et al. IL-6 trans-signaling increases expression of airways disease genes in airway smooth muscle. American Journal of Physiology - Lung Cellular and Molecular Physiology. 2015;**309**(2):L129-LL38

[3] Ye YL, Wu HT, Lin CF, Hsieh CY, Wang JY, Liu FH, et al. Dermatophagoides pteronyssinus 2 regulates nerve growth factor release to induce airway inflammation via a reactive oxygen species-dependent pathway. American Journal of Physiology. Lung Cellular and Molecular Physiology. 2011;**300**(2):L216-L224

[4] Redhu N, Gounni A. Function and mechanisms of TSLP/TSLPR complex in asthma and COPD. Clinical & Experimental Allergy. 2012;**42**(7):994-1005

[5] Redhu NS, Saleh A, Halayko AJ, Ali AS, Gounni AS. Essential role of NF-κB and AP-1 transcription factors in TNF-α-induced TSLP expression in human airway smooth muscle cells. American Journal of Physiology - Lung Cellular and Molecular Physiology. 2010;**300**(3):L479-LL85

[6] Damera G, Tliba O, Panettieri RA Jr. Airway smooth muscle as an immunomodulatory cell. Pulmonary Pharmacology & Therapeutics. 2009;**22**(5):353-359

[7] Alrashdan YA, Alkhouri H, Chen E, Lalor DJ, Poniris M, Henness S, et al. Asthmatic airway smooth muscle CXCL10 production: Mitogen-activated protein kinase JNK involvement. American Journal of Physiology - Lung Cellular and Molecular Physiology. 2012;**302**(10):L1118-L1L27

[8] Tan X, Alrashdan YA, Alkhouri H, Oliver BG, Armour CL, Hughes JM. Airway smooth muscle CXCR3 ligand production: Regulation by JAK-STAT1 and intracellular Ca2+. American Journal of Physiology - Lung Cellular and Molecular Physiology. 2013;**304**(11):L790-L802

[9] Aravamudan B, Thompson M, Pabelick C, Prakash Y. Brain-derived neurotrophic factor induces proliferation of human airway smooth muscle cells. Journal of Cellular and Molecular Medicine. 2012;**16**(4):812-823

[10] Hirota N, Martin JG. Mechanisms of airway remodeling. Chest. 2013;**144**(3):1026-1032

[11] Churg A, Zhou S, Wright JL. Series "matrix metalloproteinases in lung health and disease": Matrix metalloproteinases in COPD. The European Respiratory Journal. 2012;**39**(1):197-209

[12] Kelly EA, Jarjour NN. Role of matrix metalloproteinases in asthma. Current Opinion in Pulmonary Medicine. 2003;**9**(1):28-33

[13] Ethell IM, Ethell DW. Matrix metalloproteinases in brain development and remodeling: Synaptic functions and targets. Journal of Neuroscience Research. 2007;**85**(13):2813-2823

[14] Xie S, Issa R, Sukkar MB, Oltmanns U, Bhavsar PK, Papi A, et al. Induction and regulation of matrix metalloproteinase-12in human airway smooth muscle cells. Respiratory Research. 2005;**6**(1):148

[15] Tran T, Teoh CM, Tam JKC, Qiao Y, Chin CY, Chong OK, et al. Laminin drives survival signals to promote a contractile smooth muscle phenotype and airway hyperreactivity. The FASEB Journal. 2013;**27**(10):3991-4003

[16] Possa SS, Charafeddine HT, Righetti RF, da Silva PA, Almeida-Reis R, Saraiva-Romanholo BM, et al. Rho-kinase inhibition attenuates airway responsiveness, inflammation, matrix remodeling, and oxidative stress activation induced by chronic inflammation. American Journal of Physiology - Lung Cellular and Molecular Physiology. 2012;**303**(11):L939-LL52

[17] Bourke JE, Li X, Foster SR, Wee E, Dagher H, Ziogas J, et al. Collagen remodelling by airway smooth muscle is resistant to steroids and β2-agonists. European Respiratory Journal. 2011;**37**(1):173-182

[18] Marchica CL, Pinelli V, Borges M, Zummer J, Narayanan V, Iozzo RV, et al. A role for decorin in a murine model of allergen-induced asthma. American Journal of Physiology - Lung Cellular and Molecular Physiology. 2011;**300**(6):L863-LL73

[19] Kuo C, Lim S, King NJ, Johnston SL, Burgess JK, Black JL, et al. Rhinovirus infection induces extracellular matrix protein deposition in asthmatic and nonasthmatic airway smooth muscle cells. American Journal of Physiology - Lung Cellular and Molecular Physiology. 2011;**300**(6):L951-L9L7

[20] Britt RD Jr, Faksh A, Vogel ER, Thompson MA, Chu V, Pandya HC, et al. Vitamin D attenuates cytokine-induced remodeling in human fetal airway smooth muscle cells. Journal of Cellular Physiology. 2015;**230**(6):1189-1198

[21] Foong RE, Bosco A, Troy NM, Gorman S, Hart PH, Kicic A, et al. Identification of genes differentially regulated by vitamin D deficiency that alter lung pathophysiology and inflammation in allergic airways disease. American Journal of Physiology - Lung Cellular and Molecular Physiology. 2016;**311**(3):L653-LL63

[22] Dekkers BG, Naeimi S, Bos IST, Menzen MH, Halayko AJ, Hashjin GS, et al. l-Thyroxine promotes a proliferative airway smooth muscle phenotype in the presence of TGF-β1. American Journal of Physiology - Lung Cellular and Molecular Physiology. 2014;**308**(3):L301-L3L6

[23] Godbole MM, Rao G, Paul B, Mohan V, Singh P, Khare D, et al. Prenatal iodine deficiency results in structurally and functionally immature lungs in neonatal rats. American Journal of Physiology - Lung Cellular and Molecular Physiology. 2012;**302**(10):L1037-L1L43

[24] Agrawal A, Mabalirajan U, Ahmad T, Ghosh B. Emerging interface between metabolic syndrome and asthma. American Journal of Respiratory Cell and Molecular Biology. 2011;**44**(3):270-275

[25] Che W, Manetsch M, Quante T, Rahman MM, Patel BS, Ge Q, et al. Sphingosine 1-phosphate induces MKP-1 expression via p38 MAPK-and CREB-mediated pathways in airway smooth muscle cells. Biochimica et Biophysica Acta - Molecular Cell Research. 2012;**1823**(10):1658-1665

[26] Che W, Parmentier J, Seidel P, Manetsch M, Ramsay EE, Alkhouri H, et al. Corticosteroids inhibit sphingosine 1-phosphate-induced interleukin-6 secretion from human airway smooth muscle via mitogen-activated protein kinase phosphatase 1-mediated repression of mitogen and stress-activated protein kinase 1. American Journal of Respiratory Cell and Molecular Biology. 2014;**50**(2):358-368

[27] Liu C, Zuo J, Pertens E, Helli PB, Janssen LJ. Regulation of rho/ROCK signaling in airway smooth muscle by membrane potential and [Ca2+] i. American Journal of Physiology - Lung Cellular and Molecular Physiology. 2005;**289**(4):L574-LL82

[28] Song T, Hao Q, Zheng Y-M, Liu Q-H, Wang Y-X. Inositol 1, 4, 5-trisphosphate activates TRPC3 channels to cause extracellular Ca2+ influx in airway smooth muscle cells. American Journal of Physiology - Lung Cellular and Molecular Physiology. 2015;**309**(12):L1455-L1L66

[29] Liu Q-H, Zheng Y-M, Wang Y-X. Two distinct signaling pathways for regulation of spontaneous local Ca2+ release by phospholipase C in airway smooth muscle cells. Pflügers Archiv - European Journal of Physiology. 2007;**453**(4):531-541

[30] Penn RB, Bond RA, Walker JK. GPCRs and arrestins in airways: Implications for asthma. In: Arrestins-Pharmacology and Therapeutic Potential. Berlin, Heidelberg: Springer; 2014. pp. 387-403

[31] Brandsma C-A, Timens W, Jonker MR, Rutgers B, Noordhoek JA, Postma DS. Differential effects of fluticasone on extracellular matrix production by airway and parenchymal fibroblasts in severe COPD. American Journal of Physiology - Lung Cellular and Molecular Physiology. 2013;**305**(8):L582-L5L9

[32] Gallos G, Townsend E, Yim P, Virag L, Zhang Y, Xu D, et al. Airway epithelium is a predominant source of endogenous airway GABA and contributes to relaxation of airway smooth muscle tone. American Journal of Physiology - Lung Cellular and Molecular Physiology. 2012;**304**(3):L191-L1L7

[33] Gallos G, Yim P, Chang S, Zhang Y, Xu D, Cook JM, et al. Targeting the restricted α-subunit repertoire of airway smooth muscle GABAA receptors augments airway smooth muscle relaxation. American Journal of Physiology - Lung Cellular and Molecular Physiology. 2011;**302**(2):L248-LL56

[34] Mizuta K, Osawa Y, Mizuta F, Xu D, Emala CW. Functional expression of GABAB receptors in airway epithelium. American Journal of Respiratory Cell and Molecular Biology. 2008;**39**(3):296-304

[35] Croasdell A, Thatcher TH, Kottmann RM, Colas RA, Dalli J, Serhan CN, et al. Resolvins attenuate inflammation and promote resolution in cigarette smoke-exposed human macrophages. American Journal of Physiology - Lung Cellular and Molecular Physiology. 2015;**309**(8):L888-L901

[36] Gallos G, Yocum GT, Siviski ME, Yim PD, Fu XW, Poe MM, et al. Selective targeting of the α5-subunit of GABAA receptors relaxes airway smooth muscle and inhibits cellular calcium handling. American Journal of Physiology - Lung Cellular and Molecular Physiology. 2015;**308**(9):L931-LL42

[37] Finney BA, Del Moral PM, Wilkinson WJ, Cayzac S, Cole M, Warburton D, et al. Regulation of mouse lung development by the extracellular calcium-sensing receptor, CaR. The Journal of Physiology. 2008;**586**(24):6007-6019

[38] Kovacs CS, Kronenberg HM. Maternal-fetal calcium and bone metabolism during pregnancy, puerperium, and lactation. Endocrine Reviews. 1997;**18**(6):832-872

[39] Yarova PL, Stewart AL, Sathish V, Britt RD, Thompson MA, Lowe AP, et al. Calcium-sensing receptor antagonists abrogate airway

hyperresponsiveness and inflammation in allergic asthma. Science Translational Medicine. 2015;7(284):284ra60-284ra60

[40] Riccardi D, Kemp PJ. The calcium-sensing receptor beyond extracellular calcium homeostasis: Conception, development, adult physiology, and disease. Annual Review of Physiology. 2012;**74**:271-297

[41] Wenzel SE, Westcott J, Smith HR, Larsen GL. Spectrum of prostanoid release after bronchoalveolar allergen challenge in atopic asthmatics and in control groups. The American Review of Respiratory Disease. 1989;**139**(450):e7

[42] Allen IC, Hartney JM, Coffman TM, Penn RB, Wess J, Koller BH. Thromboxane A2 induces airway constriction through an M3 muscarinic acetylcholine receptor-dependent mechanism. American Journal of Physiology - Lung Cellular and Molecular Physiology. 2006;**290**(3):L526-LL33

[43] Deshpande DA, Wang WC, McIlmoyle EL, Robinett KS, Schillinger RM, An SS, et al. Bitter taste receptors on airway smooth muscle bronchodilate by localized calcium signaling and reverse obstruction. Nature Medicine. 2010;**16**(11):1299

[44] Robinett KS, Deshpande DA, Malone MM, Liggett SB. Agonist-promoted homologous desensitization of human airway smooth muscle bitter taste receptors. American Journal of Respiratory Cell and Molecular Biology. 2011;**45**(5):1069-1074

[45] Zhang T, Luo X-J, Sai W-B, Yu M-F, Li W-E, Ma Y-F, et al. Non-selective cation channels mediate chloroquine-induced relaxation in precontracted mouse airway smooth muscle. PLoS One. 2014;**9**(7):e101578

[46] Pulkkinen V, Manson ML, Säfholm J, Adner M, Dahlén S-E. The bitter taste receptor (TAS2R) agonists denatonium and chloroquine display distinct patterns of relaxation of the Guinea pig trachea. American Journal of Physiology - Lung Cellular and Molecular Physiology. 2012;**303**(11):L956-LL66

[47] Zhang C-H, Lifshitz LM, Uy KF, Ikebe M, Fogarty KE, ZhuGe R. The cellular and molecular basis of bitter tastant-induced bronchodilation. PLoS Biology. 2013;**11**(3):e1001501

[48] An SS, Wang WC, Koziol-White CJ, Ahn K, Lee DY, Kurten RC, et al. TAS2R activation promotes airway smooth muscle relaxation despite β2-adrenergic receptor tachyphylaxis. American Journal of Physiology - Lung Cellular and Molecular Physiology. 2012;**303**(4):L304-LL11

[49] Shaik FA, Singh N, Arakawa M, Duan K, Bhullar RP, Chelikani P. Bitter taste receptors: Extraoral roles in pathophysiology. The International Journal of Biochemistry & Cell Biology. 2016;**77**:197-204

[50] Claar D, Hartert TV, Peebles RS Jr. The role of prostaglandins in allergic lung inflammation and asthma. Expert Review of Respiratory Medicine. 2015;**9**(1):55-72

[51] Aso H, Ito S, Mori A, Suganuma N, Morioka M, Takahara N, et al. Differential regulation of airway smooth muscle cell migration by E-prostanoid receptor subtypes. American Journal of Respiratory Cell and Molecular Biology. 2013;**48**(3):322-329

[52] Kumawat K, Menzen MH, Bos IST, Baarsma HA, Borger P, Roth M, et al. Noncanonical WNT-5A signaling regulates TGF-β-induced extracellular matrix production by airway smooth muscle cells. The FASEB Journal. 2013;**27**(4):1631-1643

[53] Zemans RL, McClendon J, Aschner Y, Briones N, Young SK, Lau LF, et al.

Role of β-catenin-regulated CCN matricellular proteins in epithelial repair after inflammatory lung injury. American Journal of Physiology - Lung Cellular and Molecular Physiology. 2013;**304**(6):L415-LL27

[54] Song T, Zheng Y-M, Vincent PA, Cai D, Rosenberg P, Wang Y-X. Canonical transient receptor potential 3 channels activate NF-κB to mediate allergic airway disease via PKC-α/IκB-α and calcineurin/IκB-β pathways. The FASEB Journal. 2015;**30**(1):214-229

[55] Maher SA, Dubuis ED, Belvisi MG. G-protein coupled receptors regulating cough. Current Opinion in Pharmacology. 2011;**11**(3):248-253

[56] Jha A, Sharma P, Anaparti V, Ryu MH, Halayko AJ. A role for transient receptor potential ankyrin 1 cation channel (TRPA1) in airway hyper-responsiveness? Canadian Journal of Physiology and Pharmacology. 2015;**93**(3):171-176

[57] Watanabe N, Horie S, Spina D, Michael GJ, Page CP, Priestley JV. Immunohistochemical localization of transient receptor potential vanilloid subtype 1 in the trachea of ovalbumin-sensitized Guinea pigs. International Archives of Allergy and Immunology. 2008;**146**(Suppl. 1):28-32

[58] McAlexander MA, Luttmann MA, Hunsberger GE, Undem BJ. Transient receptor potential vanilloid 4 activation constricts the human bronchus via the release of cysteinyl leukotrienes. Journal of Pharmacology and Experimental Therapeutics. 2014;**349**(1):118-125

[59] Zhao L, Sullivan MN, Chase M, Gonzales AL, Earley S. Calcineurin/nuclear factor of activated T cells-coupled vanilliod transient receptor potential channel 4 Ca2+ sparklets stimulate airway smooth muscle cell proliferation. American Journal of Respiratory Cell and Molecular Biology. 2014;**50**(6):1064-1075

[60] Nassini R, Pedretti P, Moretto N, Fusi C, Carnini C, Facchinetti F, et al. Transient receptor potential ankyrin 1 channel localized to non-neuronal airway cells promotes non-neurogenic inflammation. PLoS One. 2012;7(8):e42454

[61] Zhang L, An X, Wang Q, He M. Activation of cold-sensitive channels TRPM8 and TRPA1 inhibits the proliferative airway smooth muscle cell phenotype. Lung. 2016;**194**(4):595-603

[62] L-m Z, Kuang H-y, L-x Z, Wu J-z, X-l C, X-y Z, et al. Effect of TRPV1 channel on proliferation and apoptosis of airway smooth muscle cells of rats. Journal of Huazhong University of Science and Technology. Medical Sciences. 2014;**34**(4):504-509

[63] Takahara N, Ito S, Furuya K, Naruse K, Aso H, Kondo M, et al. Real-time imaging of ATP release induced by mechanical stretch in human airway smooth muscle cells. American Journal of Respiratory Cell and Molecular Biology. 2014;**51**(6):772-782

[64] Siddiqui S, Novali M, Tsuchiya K, Hirota N, Geller BJ, McGovern TK, et al. The modulation of large airway smooth muscle phenotype and effects of epidermal growth factor receptor inhibition in the repeatedly allergen-challenged rat. American Journal of Physiology - Lung Cellular and Molecular Physiology. 2013;**304**(12):L853-LL62

[65] Lauer ME, Cheng G, Swaidani S, Aronica MA, Weigel PH, Hascall VC. Tumor necrosis factor-stimulated gene-6 (TSG-6) amplifies hyaluronan synthesis by airway smooth muscle cells. Journal of Biological Chemistry. 2013;**288**(1):423-431

[66] Garantziotis S, Brezina M, Castelnuovo P, Drago L. The role of hyaluronan in the pathobiology and treatment of respiratory disease.

American Journal of Physiology - Lung Cellular and Molecular Physiology. 2016;**310**(9):L785-LL95

[67] Darby PJ, Kwan C, Daniel EE. Caveolae from canine airway smooth muscle contain the necessary components for a role in Ca2+ handling. American Journal of Physiology - Lung Cellular and Molecular Physiology. 2000;**279**(6):L1226-L1L35

[68] Prakash Y, Thompson MA, Vaa B, Matabdin I, Peterson TE, He T, et al. Caveolins and intracellular calcium regulation in human airway smooth muscle. American Journal of Physiology - Lung Cellular and Molecular Physiology. 2007;**293**(5):L1118-L1L26

[69] Sathish V, Abcejo AJ, VanOosten SK, Thompson MA, Prakash Y, Pabelick CM. Caveolin-1 in cytokine-induced enhancement of intracellular Ca2+ in human airway smooth muscle. American Journal of Physiology - Lung Cellular and Molecular Physiology. 2011;**301**(4):L607-LL14

[70] Gosens R, Stelmack GL, Bos ST, Dueck G, Mutawe MM, Schaafsma D, et al. Caveolin-1 is required for contractile phenotype expression by airway smooth muscle cells. Journal of Cellular and Molecular Medicine. 2011;**15**(11):2430-2442

[71] Benayoun L, Druilhe A, Dombret M-C, Aubier M, Pretolani M. Airway structural alterations selectively associated with severe asthma. American Journal of Respiratory and Critical Care Medicine. 2003;**167**(10):1360-1368

[72] Shiomi T, Tschumperlin DJ, Park J-A, Sunnarborg SW, Horiuchi K, Blobel CP, et al. TNF-α-converting enzyme/a disintegrin and metalloprotease-17 mediates mechanotransduction in murine tracheal epithelial cells. American Journal of Respiratory Cell and Molecular Biology. 2011;**45**(2):376-385

[73] Kwak HJ, Park DW, Seo J-Y, Moon J-Y, Kim TH, Sohn JW, et al. The Wnt/β-catenin signaling pathway regulates the development of airway remodeling in patients with asthma. Experimental & Molecular Medicine. 2015;**47**(12):e198

[74] Zhou L, Goldsmith AM, Bentley JK, Jia Y, Rodriguez ML, Abe MK, et al. 4E-binding protein phosphorylation and eukaryotic initiation factor-4E release are required for airway smooth muscle hypertrophy. American Journal of Respiratory Cell and Molecular Biology. 2005;**33**(2):195-202

[75] Trian T, Benard G, Begueret H, Rossignol R, Girodet P-O, Ghosh D, et al. Bronchial smooth muscle remodeling involves calcium-dependent enhanced mitochondrial biogenesis in asthma. Journal of Experimental Medicine. 2007;**204**(13):3173-3181

[76] Pieper M, Chaudhary N, Park J. Acetylcholine-induced proliferation of fibroblasts and myofibroblasts in vitro is inhibited by tiotropium bromide. Life Sciences. 2007;**80**(24-25):2270-2273

[77] Dekkers BG, Maarsingh H, Meurs H, Gosens R. Airway structural components drive airway smooth muscle remodeling in asthma. Proceedings of the American Thoracic Society. 2009;**6**(8):683-692

[78] Simeone-Penney MC, Severgnini M, Rozo L, Takahashi S, Cochran BH, Simon AR. PDGF-induced human airway smooth muscle cell proliferation requires STAT3 and the small GTPase Rac1. American Journal of Physiology - Lung Cellular and Molecular Physiology. 2008;**294**(4):L698-L704

[79] Townsend EA, Miller VM, Prakash Y. Sex differences and sex steroids in lung health and disease. Endocrine Reviews. 2012;**33**(1):1-47

[80] Larner-Svensson HM, Williams AE, Tsitsiou E, Perry MM, Jiang X, Chung

KF, et al. Pharmacological studies of the mechanism and function of interleukin-1β-induced miRNA-146a expression in primary human airway smooth muscle. Respiratory Research. 2010;**11**(1):68

[81] Schuliga M, Ong SC, Soon L, Zal F, Harris T, Stewart AG. Airway smooth muscle remodels pericellular collagen fibrils: Implications for proliferation. American Journal of Physiology - Lung Cellular and Molecular Physiology. 2010;**298**(4):L584-LL92

[82] Billington CK, Ojo OO, Penn RB, Ito S. cAMP regulation of airway smooth muscle function. Pulmonary Pharmacology & Therapeutics. 2013;**26**(1):112-120

[83] Donovan C, Tan X, Bourke JE. PPARγ ligands regulate noncontractile and contractile functions of airway smooth muscle: Implications for asthma therapy. PPAR Research. 2012;**2012**:809164

[84] Halwani R, Al-Abri J, Beland M, Al-Jahdali H, Halayko AJ, Lee TH, et al. CC and CXC chemokines induce airway smooth muscle proliferation and survival. The Journal of Immunology. 2011:1001210

[85] Ghavami S, Mutawe MM, Schaafsma D, Yeganeh B, Unruh H, Klonisch T, et al. Geranylgeranyl transferase 1 modulates autophagy and apoptosis in human airway smooth muscle. American Journal of Physiology - Lung Cellular and Molecular Physiology. 2011;**302**(4):L420-L4L8

[86] Fogli S, Stefanelli F, Picchianti L, Del Re M, Mey V, Bardelli C, et al. Synergistic interaction between PPAR ligands and salbutamol on human bronchial smooth muscle cell proliferation. British Journal of Pharmacology. 2013;**168**(1):266-275

[87] Folinsbee LJ. Human health effects of exposure to airborne acid. Environmental Health Perspectives. 1989;**79**:195

[88] Jyothula SS, Eissa NT. Autophagy and role in asthma. Current Opinion in Pulmonary Medicine. 2013;**19**(1):30-35

[89] Poon A, Eidelman D, Laprise C, Hamid Q. ATG5, autophagy and lung function in asthma. Autophagy. 2012;**8**(4):694-695

[90] Williams AE, Larner-Svensson H, Perry MM, Campbell GA, Herrick SE, Adcock IM, et al. MicroRNA expression profiling in mild asthmatic human airways and effect of corticosteroid therapy. PLoS One. 2009;**4**(6):e5889

[91] Comer BS, Camoretti-Mercado B, Kogut PC, Halayko AJ, Solway J, Gerthoffer WT. MicroRNA-146a and microRNA-146b expression and anti-inflammatory function in human airway smooth muscle. American Journal of Physiology - Lung Cellular and Molecular Physiology. 2014;**307**(9):L727-LL34

[92] Jude JA, Dileepan M, Subramanian S, Solway J, Panettieri RA Jr, Walseth TF, et al. miR-140-3p regulation of TNF-α-induced CD38 expression in human airway smooth muscle cells. American Journal of Physiology - Lung Cellular and Molecular Physiology. 2012;**303**(5):L460-L4L8

[93] Deshpande D, Dileepan M, Walseth T, Subramanian S, Kannan M. MicroRNA regulation of airway inflammation and airway smooth muscle function: Relevance to asthma. Drug Development Research. 2015;**76**(6):286-295

[94] Dileepan M, Jude JA, Rao SP, Walseth TF, Panettieri RA, Subramanian S, et al. MicroRNA-708 regulates CD38 expression through signaling pathways JNK MAP kinase and PTEN/AKT in human airway smooth muscle cells. Respiratory Research. 2014;**15**(1):107

[95] Guedes AG, Deshpande DA, Dileepan M, Walseth TF, Panettieri RA Jr, Subramanian S, et al. CD38 and airway hyper-responsiveness: Studies on human airway smooth muscle cells and mouse models. Canadian Journal of Physiology and Pharmacology. 2014;**93**(2):145-153

[96] Mohamed JS, Hajira A, Li Z, Paulin D, Boriek AM. Desmin regulates airway smooth muscle hypertrophy through early growth-responsive protein-1 and microRNA-26a. Journal of Biological Chemistry. 2011;**286**(50):43394-43404

[97] Hu R, Pan W, Fedulov AV, Jester W, Jones MR, Weiss ST, et al. MicroRNA-10a controls airway smooth muscle cell proliferation via direct targeting of the PI3 kinase pathway. The FASEB Journal. 2014;**28**(5):2347-2357

[98] Chen M, Huang L, Zhang W, Shi J, Lin X, Lv Z, et al. MiR-23b controls TGF-β1 induced airway smooth muscle cell proliferation via TGFβR2/p-Smad3 signals. Molecular Immunology. 2016;**70**:84-93

[99] Liu Y, Yang K, Sun X, Fang P, Shi H, Xu J, et al. MiR-138 suppresses airway smooth muscle cell proliferation through the PI3K/AKT signaling pathway by targeting PDK1. Experimental Lung Research. 2015;**41**(7):363-369

[100] Liu Y, Sun X, Wu Y, Fang P, Shi H, Xu J, et al. Effects of miRNA-145 on airway smooth muscle cells function. Molecular and Cellular Biochemistry. 2015;**409**(1-2):135-143

[101] Liao G, Panettieri RA, Tang DD. MicroRNA-203 negatively regulates c-Abl, ERK1/2 phosphorylation, and proliferation in smooth muscle cells. Physiological Reports. 2015;**3**(9):e12541

[102] Aravamudan B, Thompson MA, Pabelick CM, Prakash Y. Mitochondria in lung diseases. Expert Review of Respiratory Medicine. 2013;**7**(6):631-646

[103] Contreras L, Drago I, Zampese E, Pozzan T. Mitochondria: The calcium connection. Biochimica et Biophysica Acta (BBA) - Bioenergetics. 2010;**1797**(6-7):607-618

[104] Rizzuto R, De Stefani D, Raffaello A, Mammucari C. Mitochondria as sensors and regulators of calcium signalling. Nature Reviews Molecular Cell Biology. 2012;**13**(9):566

[105] Girodet P-O, Allard B, Thumerel M, Begueret H, Dupin I, Ousova O, et al. Bronchial smooth muscle remodeling in nonsevere asthma. American Journal of Respiratory and Critical Care Medicine. 2016;**193**(6):627-633

[106] Chen T, Zhu L, Wang T, Ye H, Huang K, Hu Q. Mitochondria depletion abolishes agonist-induced Ca2+ plateau in airway smooth muscle cells: Potential role of H2O2. American Journal of Physiology - Lung Cellular and Molecular Physiology. 2009;**298**(2):L178-LL88

[107] Michaeloudes C, Sukkar MB, Khorasani NM, Bhavsar PK, Chung KF. TGF-β regulates Nox4, MnSOD and catalase expression, and IL-6 release in airway smooth muscle cells. American Journal of Physiology - Lung Cellular and Molecular Physiology. 2010;**300**(2):L295-L304

[108] Delmotte P, Sieck GC. Interaction between endoplasmic/sarcoplasmic reticulum stress (ER/SR stress), mitochondrial signaling and Ca2+ regulation in airway smooth muscle (ASM). Canadian Journal of Physiology and Pharmacology. 2014;**93**(2):97-110

[109] Guo Q, Li H, Liu J, Xu L, Yang L, Sun Z, et al. Tunicamycin aggravates endoplasmic reticulum stress and airway inflammation via PERK-ATF4-CHOP signaling in a murine model of

neutrophilic asthma. Journal of Asthma. 2017;**54**(2):125-133

[110] Hsu KJ, Turvey SE. Functional analysis of the impact of ORMDL3 expression on inflammation and activation of the unfolded protein response in human airway epithelial cells. Allergy, Asthma & Clinical Immunology. 2013;**9**(1):4

Chapter 4

Endothelial Cells in Asthma

Andrew Reichard and Kewal Asosingh

Abstract

The occurrence of new blood vessel formation in the airway wall of asthma patients was reported more than a century ago. It was long thought that angiogenesis in asthma was an epiphenomenon of airway inflammation. Therefore, little research has been performed on the role of endothelial cells in this disease. We are moving away from this misconception as an increasing number of clinical studies and findings in murine models of asthma demonstrate a causal link between angiogenesis in the airway and genesis of allergic asthma. In this chapter, we review the evidence supporting key roles for the endothelium and other angiogenic cells in the pathogenesis of asthma.

Keywords: endothelium, angiogenesis, VEGF, inflammation, PACs, Th2

1. Introduction

Allergic asthma is a chronic inflammatory disease of the conducting airways. The incidence of asthma is steadily increasing, and it has become a major health problem worldwide. The disease presents with airway inflammation, bronchoconstriction, and remodeling of the airway wall including mucus or goblet cell metaplasia, airway fibrosis, increased microvascular permeability, and angiogenesis [1].

Generally, blood vessels exhibit a two-part response upon tissue inflammation. In the first phase, which lasts about 24 hours, functional changes occur in existing blood vessels as endothelial cells are activated and vessel permeability increases. Following this initial phase, vessel remodeling and angiogenesis occur, ensuring adequate blood and nutrient delivery to tissues for survival [2–4]. When inflammation becomes chronic, immune and inflammatory cells continually infiltrate tissues, causing simultaneous damage and repair and allowing the angiogenic response to become permanent [2, 5, 6].

Chronic inflammation and the associated angiogenic response play a role in several inflammatory diseases. For example, in inflammatory bowel disease (IBD), continuous ulceration and regeneration in the bowel rely on immune-driven angiogenesis which leads to the enhanced microvessel density associated with IBD [7, 8]. Psoriatic arthritis presents with torturous, elongated blood vessels along with an increase in the number of blood vessels of the synovial membrane, contributing to the joint inflammation which is a hallmark of the disease [9]. Rheumatoid arthritis also presents with increased vascularity and inflammation of the synovial membrane due to angiogenesis, but blood vessels exhibit normal branching and structure [10]. In cancer, tumors require angiogenesis in order to continue growth and are not hindered by the disorganized, leaky, torturous vessels that result from the associated inflammation [11].

Over a century ago, researchers first observed the presence of excess small blood vessels crowded closely together in the asthmatic airway. These early studies aimed to determine the pathology of asthma and involved examining ejected sputum from asthmatic patients and extracted lungs from patients post mortem following sudden asphyxic asthma death (SAAD), or death by asthma attack. In addition to finding excess small blood vessels, these early studies also showed thickening and scarring of the bronchial wall, accumulation of leukocytes and eosinophils in the asthmatic airway, and the formation of dense, mucus-filled plugs or blockages in the lumen of the airway [12]. A subsequent study identified a dense exudate located in the bronchial lumen, likely similar to those masses observed a half century earlier, containing accumulations of eosinophils which were recruited to the airway [13]. This study also uncovered other features now firmly associated with angiogenesis and asthma, including dilated capillary blood vessels and swollen, activated endothelial cells. Around the same time, allergic inflammation in the asthmatic airway was also found to contribute to the formation of the dense exudate along with vessel engorgement, dilation, and permeability [14, 15]. Since these seminal studies, it has become well established that along with these symptoms, asthma presents with angiogenic remodeling of the vascular bed throughout the bronchial wall [1, 16]. Another study reported that angiogenesis is initiated in the early phases of adult asthma, suggesting that this process may play a role in the genesis of the disease [17].

Like in any other inflammatory diseases, the airway endothelium plays a classical role in asthmatic airway inflammation by recruiting inflammatory cells. Angiogenesis exacerbates this inflammatory response by facilitating the influx of inflammatory cells to the lungs through the newly formed blood vessels, and the permeability of these new vessels contributes to airway edema due to vessel leak [18–21]. Inflammatory cells arriving in the lungs migrate through the endothelial layer into the airway walls and induce tissue damage via the release of various mediators [22]. When specific endothelial cell adhesion molecules are lacking, inflammatory cell influx into the lungs decreases, resulting in reduced transendothelial migration and a reduction of airway hyperresponsiveness [23]. Thus, the surface receptors of endothelial cells in the lungs are a potential target for preventing airway inflammation and bronchoconstriction. This review is focused on angiogenic mechanisms in asthma, beyond their classical roles in the recruitment of immune cells.

2. Angiogenesis and its mechanism relevant to asthma

Neovascularization is the formation of new blood vessels, including vasculogenesis, arteriogenesis, and angiogenesis [1, 24, 25]. Angiogenesis is the formation of new blood vessels as an extension of pre-existing vessels. Under conditions of homeostasis, a balance exists between angiogenic activators and inhibitors, and a state of vascular quiescence is maintained in which there is no net change in vascularization [1].

Patients with asthma are no longer maintaining vascular quiescence in the bronchial wall and thus have reached a pro-angiogenic state. This pathological angiogenesis occurs due to overproduction of angiogenic factors, underproduction of inhibitors, or a combination of each of these issues, leading to increased vascularization [1]. Increased numbers of blood vessels in the bronchial wall is strongly correlated to the severity of asthma [19–21]. Increased vascularity in the airway and the increased vessel permeability which occurs concurrently contribute to the thickening of the inner airway wall and the development of airway edema [18, 19]. These symptoms lead to narrowing of the airway lumen which reduces airflow and leads to the obstructive symptoms of asthma [18–21, 26]. In healthy patients, airway smooth muscles contract, causing the luminal boundary to buckle. The luminal wall conforms to a distinct folding pattern which allows normal lung function. When the airway wall thickens as a result of asthma, fewer luminal folds are able to form upon contraction and buckling, leading to the airway obstruction observed in asthmatic patients [27].

The most studied angiogenic factor associated with increased airway vascularity in asthma is vascular endothelial growth factor (VEGF) [28]. Angiogenesis is dependent upon VEGF and its tyrosine kinase receptors (VEGFR) [29]. The VEGF family consists of VEGF-A, VEGF-B, VEGF-C, VEGF-D, and placental growth factor (PlGF) [30]. The members of the VEGF family bind to one or multiple types of VEGFR, which are denoted as VEGFR-1, VEGFR-2, and VEGFR-3 [30]. Each VEGFR is predominantly expressed on specific cell types: VEGFR-1 on monocytes and macrophages, VEGFR-2 on vascular endothelial cells, and VEGFR-3 on lymphatic endothelial cells and endothelial cells of sprouting blood vessels [31]. However, each receptor type plays multiple roles in angiogenesis and other processes through lower level expression on other cell types and through binding multiple ligands of the VEGF family. VEGFR-1, the only receptor which binds PlGF and VEGF-B, plays a role in controlling angiogenesis through functions associated with both endothelial and non-endothelial cells [32]. VEGFR-1 and VEGFR-2 both bind to VEGF-A, which is the prototypical member of the VEGF family and is often denoted as simply VEGF [32]. VEGFR-2 has been shown to be the primary mitogenic receptor for VEGF in the angiogenesis pathway, binding VEGF which has been released by nearby tissues in a paracrine fashion [33, 34]. VEGFR-2 and VEGFR-3 each bind to VEGF-C and VEGF-D, inducing angiogenic and lymphangiogenic activity [32]. It is important to note that VEGF-C, while commonly viewed as controlling lymphangiogenesis specifically, can also induce blood vessel angiogenesis by stimulating endothelial cell migration and proliferation when binding to VEGFR-3 on blood vessel endothelial cells [35–38]. Blocking VEGFR-3 through specific antagonistic antibodies has been shown to decrease the number of proliferating endothelial cells, directly linking this receptor to angiogenesis [39]. VEGF is also responsible for activating the extracellular signal-regulated kinase (ERK) pathway [40]. The ERK pathway helps to control migration, proliferation, and apoptosis of endothelial cells and therefore plays a significant role in angiogenesis [41].

Two cell types directly involved in angiogenesis are pro-angiogenic hematopoietic progenitor cells and endothelial colony-forming cells. Pro-angiogenic hematopoietic progenitor cells (PACs) are a heterogeneous population of cells serving in a paracrine function to promote angiogenic activity. This heterogeneous population of pro-angiogenic cells is made up of subsets of hematopoietic progenitor cells but can also include mature blood cells such as monocytes [42–45]. The hematopoietic stem or progenitor cells are typically committed to the myeloid lineage and stimulate local angiogenic responses through a paracrine release of growth factors [46–50]. PACs are known to play a significant role in asthma due to their pro-angiogenic activity [49, 51–55]. Endothelial colony-forming cells (ECFCs), sometimes referred to as late outgrowth endothelial cells (OECs), are true endothelial cell precursors which proliferate to form new blood vessels as part of the angiogenic process [42–45, 56]. ECFCs are rare in circulation but incorporate into existing microvessels, functioning as the building blocks of new vasculature by dividing and proliferating quickly [1, 46–48, 57]. ECFCs and PACs participate synergistically in the process of neovascularization, and both cell types are required in an angiogenic response [58]. These two cell types were originally collectively referred to as endothelial progenitor cells (EPCs) [59]. However, it became apparent that a variety of blood and endothelial cells were being grouped together under this umbrella term [60, 61]. The lineage relationships among EPCs that led to their suggested reclassification and the removal of this umbrella term have been reviewed [42]. PACs and ECFCs do in fact share a common embryonic origin, the hemangioblast, which is capable of developing into both hematopoietic and endothelial precursor cells [62]. Hemangioblasts have been shown to play a significant role in embryologic development as bipotent stem cells and have recently been found to remain active during adult development, most notably in the bone marrow [62]. It has been proposed that the synergy and dependence between PACs and ECFCs observed in angiogenesis are a result of the common developmental origin of the vascular and hematopoietic system, centered on the hemangioblast [26]. PACs and ECFCs also share similar functions, cell markers, and in vitro phenotypes, again most likely stemming from their common origin [26]. However, more recent analysis has revealed that PACs are in fact hematopoietic cells derived from the bone marrow which differ from the ECFCs studied in angiogenesis [42, 49, 56, 63, 64]. This leads us to the current classification used to distinguish the two cooperating but distinct cell types involved in asthma-related angiogenesis.

Recruitment of PACs into the lungs is an early step in initiating airway wall angiogenesis in asthma. C-X-C motif chemokine receptor 2 (CXCR2) and C-X-C motif chemokine receptor 4 (CXCR4) are important receptors in inflammatory and angiogenic pathways [55, 65, 66]. CXCR2 and CXCR4 are expressed by PACs and vascular endothelial cells and are activated by one of eight known ligands [54, 56]. These ligands are released within hours of lung allergen exposure and act as chemoattractants to promote the activation and lung-homing of PACs [54, 55]. The accumulation of PACs in the lungs and perivascular tissue promotes inflammation and accumulates VEGF, leading to increased angiogenesis [67–69]. Blocking CXCR2 receptors has been shown to reduce the accumulation of PACs in the lungs and the occurrence of airway angiogenesis, proving the essential nature of recruiting PACs in the angiogenic pathway [70].

Another receptor that has been shown to play a pivotal role in pathological angiogenesis is C-C motif chemokine receptor 3 (CCR3). CCR3 is expressed by angiogenic endothelial cells and eosinophils and acts as a receptor for eotaxin [53, 71–73]. Eotaxin is a chemokine expressed by endothelial cells, epithelial cells, and PACs, among others, and presents at particularly high levels in the lung endothelium in asthmatic patients and allergen-exposed mice [53]. Eotaxins have traditionally been known to act as the major chemoattractant of eosinophils, which contribute to the airway inflammation in allergic asthma. Asthmatic patients are therefore known to express higher levels of eotaxins [52]. However, eotaxins have also been shown to induce migration and angiogenic tube formation by CCR3-expressing lung endothelial cells [72]. This confirms the role of eotaxins as major angiogenic factors, alongside VEGF, contributing to airway remodeling in allergic asthma.

3. Animal models

Murine models are utilized to study the underlying mechanisms of asthma and to conduct preclinical testing of novel therapeutic strategies. Allergen exposure in murine models allows the induction of an allergic response in a controlled setting that is meant to resemble the symptoms of asthma seen in patients. This is an insightful alternative to observing established asthma in clinical studies. Two common murine models of allergic asthma used in research are the house dust mite extract (HDME) model and the ovalbumin (OVA) model [52, 74–76].

Experiments in the OVA model showed that chronic allergen exposure induces mobilization and lung-homing of PACs, increasing vascularity of the airway wall through angiogenesis, endothelial activation, and airway resistance within hours of allergen exposure [51–55, 77]. Blocking CXCR4 resulted in reduced lung-homing of PACs along with reduced airway inflammation and airway hyperresponsiveness, blunting the effects of OVA challenge [55]. Type 2 helper (Th2) cells are immune cells which contribute to the Th2-mediated inflammatory response in asthma following allergen challenge by promoting eosinophilia and stimulating the production of specific cytokines involved in asthma pathogenesis [78–80]. These Th2 cells cooperate with type 1 helper (Th1) cells to contribute to the asthmatic phenotype [16, 81–83]. OVA challenge induces angiogenesis, promoting the Th2 inflammatory response, also known as the type 2 immune response, through the production of pro-Th2 cytokines. Interleukin-25 (IL-25), also known as IL-17E, is an upstream master regulator of Th2-mediated inflammation [84–88]. IL-25 is expressed by various cell types, including epithelial and endothelial cells, mast cells, T cells, and eosinophils [84, 88–93]. It was recently shown that endothelial cells facilitate the type 2 immune response in asthma by producing IL-25. Th2 activation complements the release of thymic stromal lymphopoietin (TSLP) by lung-recruited PACs [51]. TSLP is a pro-Th2 cytokine expressed in endothelial cells, epithelial cells, neutrophils, macrophages, and mast cells which plays a role in the maturation of T cells and eosinophils [94, 95]. The combined effects of IL-25 and TSLP contribute to angiogenesis and eosinophilia by inducing the expression of eotaxins by PACs and other cell types [53].

More recent studies have utilized the HDME model, which is clinically relevant as house dust mite allergens are a potent inducer of asthma worldwide [96]. HDME-exposed mice present with increased accumulation of PACs, increased vascularity of the airway, airway inflammation, and airway hyperresponsiveness [77, 97]. VEGFR-3 and its ligand VEGF-C are critical in new vessel sprouting in asthmatic angiogenesis [97]. VEGFR-3 is expressed exclusively in blood vessels actively undergoing angiogenesis, and this VEGFR-3 expression is known to increase when cells are exposed to HDME [97]. HDME exposure promotes differentiation and proliferation of PACs, induces secretion of VEGF-C, and upregulates protease-activated receptor 2 (PAR-2) [97–102]. PAR-2 is a key house dust mite allergen-sensing receptor mainly expressed on airway epithelial cells, endothelial cells, and dendritic cells [103–109]. PAR-2 initiates the Th2 inflammatory responses to HDME and is also an important regulator of angiogenesis [98, 99, 110]. House dust mite proteases penetrate deep into the airway mucosa, activating endothelial cells via PAR-2 and triggering the onset of angiogenesis in the airway [97]. This endothelial activation of PAR-2 induces the production of pro-Th2 cytokines including interleukin-1α (IL-1α) and granulocyte-macrophage colony-stimulating factor (GM-CSF) [109, 111–113]. IL-1α activates dendritic cells and controls the Th2 inflammatory response by inducing release of GM-CSF and TSLP by other cells [113]. GM-CSF activates dendritic cells which stimulate Th2 cells [113–118]. Together, these results show that house dust mite proteases induce angiogenesis, airway inflammation, and airway hyperresponsiveness through the activation of endothelial cells, mobilization of PACs, and upregulation of VEGFR-3 and VEGF-C.

The timeline of the progression and development of angiogenesis has also been studied in murine asthma models. PACs are recruited to the lungs within a few hours of allergen challenge, creating a pro-angiogenic environment in the lungs within 48 hours. However, the influx of inflammatory cells, namely, eosinophils, observed in the asthmatic airway following allergen challenge does not reach its peak until 4–6 days after allergen challenge [16]. This indicates that angiogenesis starts in the lungs before bulk inflammation occurs, suggesting that endothelial cell activation in asthma occurs independently of inflammation and reinforcing the importance of researching the angiogenic mechanisms in asthma. Other reports confirmed that PAC recruitment and neovascularization occur prior to airway inflammation [1, 119].

Recent research has focused on developing strategies to inhibit angiogenesis in the lungs as a novel therapeutic approach in asthma. Targeting PACs has proven to be an effective method of controlling angiogenesis in the asthmatic airway in a murine model. AMD3100, a chemokine receptor antagonist, was administered to mice during OVA allergen challenge. Accumulation of PACs in the airway was attenuated, as was eosinophilic inflammation, airway hyperresponsiveness, and airway vascularity due to the mitigation of angiogenesis [55]. Mice with established asthma symptoms that were treated with AMD3100 exhibited only partially reversed airway hyperresponsiveness despite the reduction of PAC and eosinophil accumulation and angiogenesis. This suggests that early detection and treatment of asthmatic angiogenesis may be crucial for clinical benefit. Drugs that prevent transendothelial migration of inflammatory cells, limiting inflammation that typically occurs in the asthmatic airway as the disease progresses, have also been explored [22]. Theophylline is an anti-inflammatory natural small molecule commonly used in asthma treatment to prevent inflammation and transendothelial migration [120]. Montelukast is a drug which serves as a leukotriene receptor antagonist, preventing the inflammatory response in the airway as well [121]. VUF-K-8788 is a histamine H1 antagonist that is able to reduce eosinophil adherence to endothelial cells in vitro while also reducing eosinophil accumulation and adherence in the airway of a guinea pig asthma model, preventing airway inflammation associated with the disease [122]. Discovering new inhibitors to target PACs and endothelial cells in the asthmatic airway will be crucial in future animal studies to explore potential therapeutic interventions for pathological angiogenesis.

4. Clinical studies

Clinical studies of patients with allergic asthma have played a key role in developing the current knowledge of neovascularization in this disease. Endobronchial biopsies are commonly performed to quantify airway inflammation and airway remodeling. A biopsy punch is used to extract tissues from the airway wall which are then studied to assess the current state of a patient's airway. For example, endobronchial biopsies have been used to compare VEGF mRNA levels in asthmatic and healthy control patients [123]. Increased VEGF mRNA indicates increased angiogenesis in asthmatic patients, as VEGF controls vascular remodeling of the airway through angiogenesis, as previously discussed. Increased VEGF mRNA levels in the airway wall may explain the elevated levels of VEGF in sputum and serum from asthmatic patients which correlate to the severity of the disease [124–129]. In another study, asthmatics presenting with airway inflammation and hyperresponsiveness underwent allergen inhalation prior to endobronchial biopsy. The endobronchial biopsy tissues showed increased presence of PACs in addition to elevated vessel numbers and size, indicative of angiogenesis [54]. Bronchoalveolar lavage (BAL) is another clinical technique used to quantify the presence of various cell types by flushing the bronchial and alveolar spaces with fluid in order to collect cells. For example, one BAL study compared the presence of PACs and total vessel density in asthmatic and healthy patients. Total vessel number was shown to be increased in the airway walls of asthma patients, as was the accumulation of PACs [17]. Increased vascularity observed in medium-sized airways in the lungs may contribute to airflow limitation, as an enhanced vascular network in the airway develops in early phases of chronic adult asthma [17].

Clinical studies of nitric oxide (NO) have also contributed to explaining endothelial cell activation in asthma. NO in circulation originates from the endothelium, while exhaled NO originates in the epithelium. When patients underwent allergen challenge by inhalation, a significant increase in serum NO levels was observed after 4 hours, while exhaled NO did not increase [53]. This indicates that endothelial cells in the airway are activated prior to epithelial cells in the airway during a controlled asthma attack induced by inhaled allergens [53]. Thus, activation of the airway endothelium is one of the earliest responses to an induced asthma attack, triggering the vascular endothelium to release NO and mobilizing PACs to initiate angiogenesis.

5. Conclusion

Despite historical studies reporting angiogenesis in asthma more than a century ago, understanding of the endothelial contribution to asthma is still in its infancy. Clinical studies show a strong correlation between neovascularization and asthma severity. Whole-lung allergen studies suggest that airway inflammation and bronchoconstriction are preceded by rapid activation of the endothelium and accompanied by mobilization and recruitment of bone marrow-derived pro-angiogenic cells into the airway, resulting in angiogenesis. Murine model studies recapitulate the clinical findings and further indicate that endothelial cells are capable of sensing allergens just as the airway epithelium and dendritic cells do. Overall, a pro-Th2 angiogenic response may have a causal role in the genesis of allergic asthma (**Figure 1**).

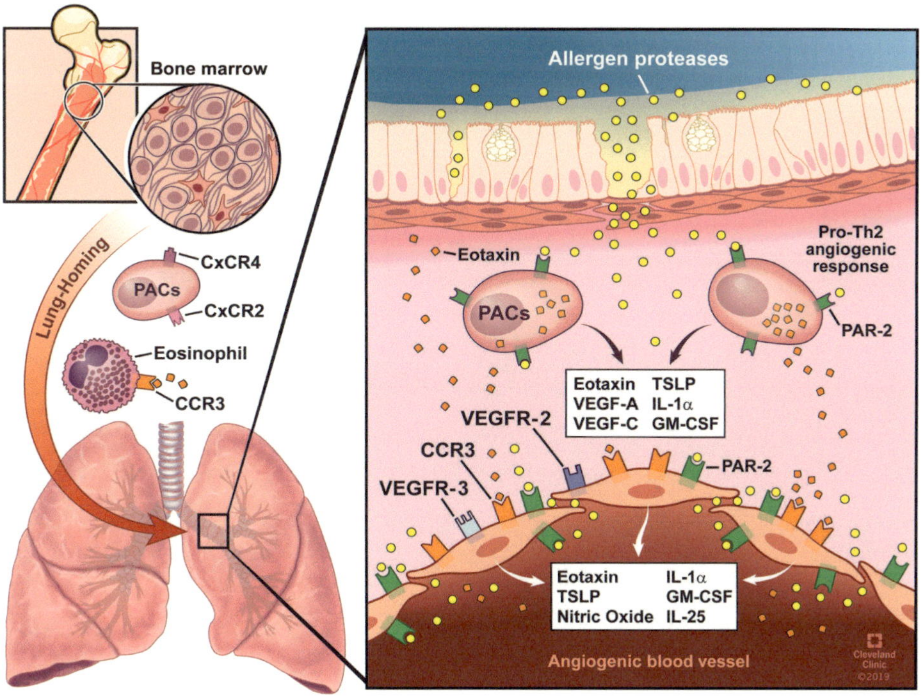

Figure 1.
Angiogenic mechanisms in asthma.

Inhaled allergen proteases breach the airway epithelial barrier allowing them to penetrate into the airway mucosa. PAR-2 expressing bone marrow-derived PACs and lung-resident endothelial cells sense the mucosal presence of house dust mite allergens and respond by releasing angiogenic factors (eotaxin, VEGF-A, VEGF-C) and Th2-promoting cytokines (TSLP, IL-1α, GM-CSF). Additional PACs expressing CXCR2 and CXCR4 receptors are recruited into the lungs. Eotaxins play a dual role by inducing angiogenesis and attracting circulating eosinophils into the lungs via CCR3 receptors. Thus, a pro-Th2 angiogenic response fuels the innate allergen sensing in the airway mucosa and promotes airway inflammation and bronchoconstriction.

Acknowledgements

The authors thank David Schumick of the Cleveland Clinic Center for Medical Art and Photography for his illustration work on **Figure 1**.

Conflict of interest

The authors declare no conflicts of interest.

Author details

Andrew Reichard and Kewal Asosingh*
Department of Inflammation and Immunity, Lerner Research Institute,
The Cleveland Clinic, Cleveland, Ohio, USA

*Address all correspondence to: asosink@ccf.org

References

[1] Asosingh K, Erzurum SC. Angioplasticity in asthma. Biochemical Society Transactions. 2009;**37**(Pt 4):805-810

[2] Majno G. Chronic inflammation: Links with angiogenesis and wound healing. The American Journal of Pathology. 1998;**153**(4):1035-1039

[3] Cines DB, Pollak ES, Buck CA, Loscalzo J, Zimmerman GA, McEver RP, et al. Endothelial cells in physiology and in the pathophysiology of vascular disorders. Blood. 1998;**91**(10):3527-3561

[4] Carmeliet P. Mechanisms of angiogenesis and arteriogenesis. Nature Medicine. 2000;**6**(4):389-395

[5] Frantz S, Vincent KA, Feron O, Kelly RA. Innate immunity and angiogenesis. Circulation Research. 2005;**96**(1):15-26

[6] Danese S, Dejana E, Fiocchi C. Immune regulation by microvascular endothelial cells: Directing innate and adaptive immunity, coagulation, and inflammation. Journal of Immunology. 2007;**178**(10):6017-6022

[7] Alkim C, Savas B, Ensari A, Alkim H, Dagli U, Parlak E, et al. Expression of p53, VEGF, microvessel density, and cyclin-D1 in noncancerous tissue of inflammatory bowel disease. Digestive Diseases and Sciences. 2009;**54**(9):1979-1984

[8] Alkim C, Alkim H, Koksal AR, Boga S, Sen I. Angiogenesis in inflammatory bowel disease. International Journal of Inflammation. 2015;**2015**:970890

[9] Cantatore FP, Maruotti N, Corrado A, Ribatti D. Angiogenesis dysregulation in psoriatic arthritis: Molecular mechanisms. BioMed Research International. 2017;**2017**:5312813

[10] Reece RJ, Canete JD, Parsons WJ, Emery P, Veale DJ. Distinct vascular patterns of early synovitis in psoriatic, reactive, and rheumatoid arthritis. Arthritis and Rheumatism. 1999;**42**(7):1481-1484

[11] Ramjiawan RR, Griffioen AW, Duda DG. Anti-angiogenesis for cancer revisited: Is there a role for combinations with immunotherapy? Angiogenesis. 2017;**20**(2):185-204

[12] Ellis AG. The pathological anatomy of bronchial asthma. The American Journal of the Medical Sciences. 1908;**186**(3):407-428

[13] Dunnill MS. The pathology of asthma, with special reference to changes in the bronchial mucosa. Journal of Clinical Pathology. 1960;**13**:27-33

[14] Segal M, Attinger E. Bronchial asthma. In: Gordon B, editor. Clinical Cardiopulmonary Physiology (American College of Chest Physicians). New York: Grune and Stratton; 1957. pp. 283-327

[15] Florey H. The secretion of mucus and inflammation of mucous membranes. In: Florey H, editor. General Pathology. 2nd ed. London: Lloyd-Luke; 1958. pp. 120-142

[16] Asosingh K, Swaidani S, Aronica M, Erzurum SC. Th1- and Th2-dependent endothelial progenitor cell recruitment and angiogenic switch in asthma. Journal of Immunology. 2007;**178**(10):6482-6494

[17] Hashimoto M, Tanaka H, Abe S. Quantitative analysis of bronchial wall vascularity in the medium and small airways of patients with asthma and COPD. Chest. 2005;**127**(3):965-972

[18] Li X, Wilson JW. Increased vascularity of the bronchial mucosa

in mild asthma. American Journal of Respiratory and Critical Care Medicine. 1997;**156**(1):229-233

[19] Salvato G. Quantitative and morphological analysis of the vascular bed in bronchial biopsy specimens from asthmatic and non-asthmatic subjects. Thorax. 2001;**56**(12):902-906

[20] Vrugt B, Wilson S, Bron A, Holgate ST, Djukanovic R, Aalbers R. Bronchial angiogenesis in severe glucocorticoid-dependent asthma. The European Respiratory Journal. 2000;**15**(6):1014-1021

[21] Pascual RM, Peters SP. Airway remodeling contributes to the progressive loss of lung function in asthma: An overview. The Journal of Allergy and Clinical Immunology. 2005;**116**(3):477-486 quiz 87

[22] Green CE, Turner AM. The role of the endothelium in asthma and chronic obstructive pulmonary disease (COPD). Respiratory Research. 2017;**18**(1):20

[23] Tang ML, Fiscus LC. Important roles for L-selectin and ICAM-1 in the development of allergic airway inflammation in asthma. Pulmonary Pharmacology & Therapeutics. 2001;**14**(3):203-210

[24] Carmeliet P. Angiogenesis in health and disease. Nature Medicine. 2003;**9**(6):653-660

[25] Semenza GL. Vasculogenesis, angiogenesis, and arteriogenesis: Mechanisms of blood vessel formation and remodeling. Journal of Cellular Biochemistry. 2007;**102**(4):840-847

[26] Duong HT, Erzurum SC, Asosingh K. Pro-angiogenic hematopoietic progenitor cells and endothelial colony-forming cells in pathological angiogenesis of bronchial and pulmonary circulation. Angiogenesis. 2011;**14**(4):411-422

[27] Wiggs BR, Hrousis CA, Drazen JM, Kamm RD. On the mechanism of mucosal folding in normal and asthmatic airways. Journal of Applied Physiology (Bethesda, MD: 1985). 1997;**83**(6):1814-1821

[28] Chetta A, Zanini A, Foresi A, D'Ippolito R, Tipa A, Castagnaro A, et al. Vascular endothelial growth factor up-regulation and bronchial wall remodelling in asthma. Clinical and Experimental Allergy. 2005;**35**(11):1437-1442

[29] Leung DW, Cachianes G, Kuang WJ, Goeddel DV, Ferrara N. Vascular endothelial growth factor is a secreted angiogenic mitogen. Science. 1989;**246**(4935):1306-1309

[30] Ferrara N, Gerber HP, LeCouter J. The biology of VEGF and its receptors. Nature Medicine. 2003;**9**(6):669-676

[31] Koch S, Tugues S, Li X, Gualandi L, Claesson-Welsh L. Signal transduction by vascular endothelial growth factor receptors. The Biochemical Journal. 2011;**437**(2):169-183

[32] Cao Y. Positive and negative modulation of angiogenesis by VEGFR1 ligands. Science Signaling. 2009;**2**(59):re1

[33] Fong GH, Rossant J, Gertsenstein M, Breitman ML. Role of the Flt-1 receptor tyrosine kinase in regulating the assembly of vascular endothelium. Nature. 1995;**376**(6535):66-70

[34] Shalaby F, Rossant J, Yamaguchi TP, Gertsenstein M, Wu XF, Breitman ML, et al. Failure of blood-island formation and vasculogenesis in Flk-1-deficient mice. Nature. 1995;**376**(6535):62-66

[35] Joukov V, Pajusola K, Kaipainen A, Chilov D, Lahtinen I, Kukk E, et al. A novel vascular endothelial growth factor, VEGF-C, is a ligand for the Flt4

(VEGFR-3) and KDR (VEGFR-2) receptor tyrosine kinases. The EMBO Journal. 1996;**15**(2):290-298

[36] Cao Y, Linden P, Farnebo J, Cao R, Eriksson A, Kumar V, et al. Vascular endothelial growth factor C induces angiogenesis in vivo. Proceedings of the National Academy of Sciences of the United States of America. 1998;**95**(24):14389-14394

[37] Witzenbichler B, Asahara T, Murohara T, Silver M, Spyridopoulos I, Magner M, et al. Vascular endothelial growth factor-C (VEGF-C/VEGF-2) promotes angiogenesis in the setting of tissue ischemia. The American Journal of Pathology. 1998;**153**(2):381-394

[38] Tammela T, Zarkada G, Nurmi H, Jakobsson L, Heinolainen K, Tvorogov D, et al. VEGFR-3 controls tip to stalk conversion at vessel fusion sites by reinforcing Notch signalling. Nature Cell Biology. 2011;**13**(10):1202-1213

[39] Tammela T, Zarkada G, Wallgard E, Murtomaki A, Suchting S, Wirzenius M, et al. Blocking VEGFR-3 suppresses angiogenic sprouting and vascular network formation. Nature. 2008;**454**(7204):656-660

[40] Wu LW, Mayo LD, Dunbar JD, Kessler KM, Baerwald MR, Jaffe EA, et al. Utilization of distinct signaling pathways by receptors for vascular endothelial cell growth factor and other mitogens in the induction of endothelial cell proliferation. The Journal of Biological Chemistry. 2000;**275**(7):5096-5103

[41] Wang S, Cao W, Xing H, Chen YL, Li Q, Shen T, et al. Activation of ERK pathway is required for 15-HETE-induced angiogenesis in human umbilical vascular endothelial cells. Journal of Receptor and Signal Transduction Research. 2016;**36**(3):225-232

[42] Richardson MR, Yoder MC. Endothelial progenitor cells: Quo vadis? Journal of Molecular and Cellular Cardiology. 2011;**50**(2):266-272

[43] Chao H, Hirschi KK. Hemato-vascular origins of endothelial progenitor cells? Microvascular Research. 2010;**79**(3):169-173

[44] Ingram DA, Mead LE, Tanaka H, Meade V, Fenoglio A, Mortell K, et al. Identification of a novel hierarchy of endothelial progenitor cells using human peripheral and umbilical cord blood. Blood. 2004;**104**(9):2752-2760

[45] Yoder MC. Defining human endothelial progenitor cells. Journal of Thrombosis and Haemostasis. 2009;**7**(Suppl 1):49-52

[46] Wilson JW, Hii S. The importance of the airway microvasculature in asthma. Current Opinion in Allergy and Clinical Immunology. 2006;**6**(1):51-55

[47] Yoder MC. Is endothelium the origin of endothelial progenitor cells? Arteriosclerosis, Thrombosis, and Vascular Biology. 2010;**30**(6):1094-1103

[48] Yoder MC, Mead LE, Prater D, Krier TR, Mroueh KN, Li F, et al. Redefining endothelial progenitor cells via clonal analysis and hematopoietic stem/progenitor cell principals. Blood. 2007;**109**(5):1801-1809

[49] Rose JA, Erzurum S, Asosingh K. Biology and flow cytometry of proangiogenic hematopoietic progenitors cells. Cytometry. Part A. 2015;**87**(1):5-19

[50] Wara AK, Croce K, Foo S, Sun X, Icli B, Tesmenitsky Y, et al. Bone marrow-derived CMPs and GMPs represent highly functional proangiogenic cells: Implications for ischemic cardiovascular disease. Blood. 2011;**118**(24):6461-6464

[51] Asosingh K, Cheng G, Xu W, Savasky BM, Aronica MA, Li X, et al. Nascent endothelium initiates Th2 polarization of asthma. Journal of Immunology. 2013;**190**(7): 3458-3465

[52] Asosingh K, Hanson JD, Cheng G, Aronica MA, Erzurum SC. Allergen-induced, eotaxin-rich, proangiogenic bone marrow progenitors: A blood-borne cellular envoy for lung eosinophilia. The Journal of Allergy and Clinical Immunology. 2010;**125**(4):918-925

[53] Asosingh K, Vasanji A, Tipton A, Queisser K, Wanner N, Janocha A, et al. Eotaxin-rich proangiogenic hematopoietic progenitor cells and CCR3+ endothelium in the atopic asthmatic response. Journal of Immunology. 2016;**196**(5):2377-2387

[54] Imaoka H, Punia N, Irshad A, Ying S, Corrigan CJ, Howie K, et al. Lung homing of endothelial progenitor cells in humans with asthma after allergen challenge. American Journal of Respiratory and Critical Care Medicine. 2011;**184**(7):771-778

[55] Doyle TM, Ellis R, Park HJ, Inman MD, Sehmi R. Modulating progenitor accumulation attenuates lung angiogenesis in a mouse model of asthma. The European Respiratory Journal. 2011;**38**(3):679-687

[56] Medina RJ, O'Neill CL, Sweeney M, Guduric-Fuchs J, Gardiner TA, Simpson DA, et al. Molecular analysis of endothelial progenitor cell (EPC) subtypes reveals two distinct cell populations with different identities. BMC Medical Genomics. 2010;**3**:18

[57] Melero-Martin JM, Khan ZA, Picard A, Wu X, Paruchuri S, Bischoff J. In vivo vasculogenic potential of human blood-derived endothelial progenitor cells. Blood. 2007;**109**(11):4761-4768

[58] Yoon CH, Hur J, Park KW, Kim JH, Lee CS, Oh IY, et al. Synergistic neovascularization by mixed transplantation of early endothelial progenitor cells and late outgrowth endothelial cells: The role of angiogenic cytokines and matrix metalloproteinases. Circulation. 2005;**112**(11):1618-1627

[59] Asahara T, Murohara T, Sullivan A, Silver M, van der Zee R, Li T, et al. Isolation of putative progenitor endothelial cells for angiogenesis. Science. 1997;**275**(5302):964-967

[60] Yoder MC, Ingram DA. Endothelial progenitor cell: Ongoing controversy for defining these cells and their role in neoangiogenesis in the murine system. Current Opinion in Hematology. 2009;**16**(4):269-273

[61] Steinmetz M, Nickenig G, Werner N. Endothelial-regenerating cells: An expanding universe. Hypertension. 2010;**55**(3):593-599

[62] Loges S, Fehse B, Brockmann MA, Lamszus K, Butzal M, Guckenbiehl M, et al. Identification of the adult human hemangioblast. Stem Cells and Development. 2004;**13**(3):229-242

[63] Rehman J, Li J, Orschell CM, March KL. Peripheral blood "endothelial progenitor cells" are derived from monocyte/macrophages and secrete angiogenic growth factors. Circulation. 2003;**107**(8):1164-1169

[64] Hur J, Yang HM, Yoon CH, Lee CS, Park KW, Kim JH, et al. Identification of a novel role of T cells in postnatal vasculogenesis: Characterization of endothelial progenitor cell colonies. Circulation. 2007;**116**(15):1671-1682

[65] Sukkar A, Jenkins J, Sanchez J, Wagner EM. Inhibition of CXCR2 attenuates bronchial angiogenesis in the ischemic rat lung. Journal of Applied

Physiology (Bethesda, MD: 1985). 2008;**104**(5):1470-1475

[66] Hristov M, Zernecke A, Bidzhekov K, Liehn EA, Shagdarsuren E, Ludwig A, et al. Importance of CXC chemokine receptor 2 in the homing of human peripheral blood endothelial progenitor cells to sites of arterial injury. Circulation Research. 2007;**100**(4):590-597

[67] Asagoe K, Yamamoto K, Takahashi A, Suzuki K, Maeda A, Nohgawa M, et al. Down-regulation of CXCR2 expression on human polymorphonuclear leukocytes by TNF-alpha. Journal of Immunology. 1998;**160**(9):4518-4525

[68] Matsuo Y, Raimondo M, Woodward TA, Wallace MB, Gill KR, Tong Z, et al. CXC-chemokine/CXCR2 biological axis promotes angiogenesis in vitro and in vivo in pancreatic cancer. International Journal of Cancer. 2009;**125**(5):1027-1037

[69] Li X, Chen Y, Chang Y, Li S, Zhao Z, Zhang H. CXCR2 is involved in pulmonary intravascular macrophage accumulation and angiogenesis in a rat model of hepatopulmonary syndrome. Clinical Science (London, England). 2017;**131**(2):159-168

[70] Jones CP, Pitchford SC, Lloyd CM, Rankin SM. CXCR2 mediates the recruitment of endothelial progenitor cells during allergic airways remodeling. Stem Cells. 2009;**27**(12):3074-3081

[71] Salcedo R, Young HA, Ponce ML, Ward JM, Kleinman HK, Murphy WJ, et al. Eotaxin (CCL11) induces in vivo angiogenic responses by human CCR3+ endothelial cells. Journal of Immunology. 2001;**166**(12):7571-7578

[72] Takeda A, Baffi JZ, Kleinman ME, Cho WG, Nozaki M, Yamada K, et al. CCR3 is a target for age-related macular degeneration diagnosis and therapy. Nature. 2009;**460**(7252):225-230

[73] Ponath PD, Qin S, Post TW, Wang J, Wu L, Gerard NP, et al. Molecular cloning and characterization of a human eotaxin receptor expressed selectively on eosinophils. The Journal of Experimental Medicine. 1996;**183**(6):2437-2448

[74] Hammad H, Plantinga M, Deswarte K, Pouliot P, Willart MA, Kool M, et al. Inflammatory dendritic cells–not basophils–are necessary and sufficient for induction of Th2 immunity to inhaled house dust mite allergen. The Journal of Experimental Medicine. 2010;**207**(10):2097-2111

[75] Plantinga M, Guilliams M, Vanheerswynghels M, Deswarte K, Branco-Madeira F, Toussaint W, et al. Conventional and monocyte-derived CD11b(+) dendritic cells initiate and maintain T helper 2 cell-mediated immunity to house dust mite allergen. Immunity. 2013;**38**(2):322-335

[76] Xu W, Ghosh S, Comhair SA, Asosingh K, Janocha AJ, Mavrakis DA, et al. Increased mitochondrial arginine metabolism supports bioenergetics in asthma. The Journal of Clinical Investigation. 2016;**126**(7):2465-2481

[77] Sivapalan N, Wattie J, Inman MD, Sehmi R. Lung-homing of endothelial progenitor cells and airway vascularization is only partially dependant on eosinophils in a house dust mite-exposed mouse model of allergic asthma. PLoS One. 2014;**9**(10):e109991

[78] Romagnani S. Th1/Th2 cells. Inflammatory Bowel Diseases. 1999;**5**(4):285-294

[79] Cazzola M, Polosa R. Anti-TNF-alpha and Th1 cytokine-directed therapies for the treatment of asthma.

Current Opinion in Allergy and Clinical Immunology. 2006;**6**(1):43-50

[80] Umetsu DT, McIntire JJ, Akbari O, Macaubas C, DeKruyff RH. Asthma: An epidemic of dysregulated immunity. Nature Immunology. 2002;**3**(8):715-720

[81] Li XM, Schofield BH, Wang QF, Kim KH, Huang SK. Induction of pulmonary allergic responses by antigen-specific Th2 cells. Journal of Immunology. 1998;**160**(3):1378-1384

[82] Randolph DA, Carruthers CJ, Szabo SJ, Murphy KM, Chaplin DD. Modulation of airway inflammation by passive transfer of allergen-specific Th1 and Th2 cells in a mouse model of asthma. Journal of Immunology. 1999;**162**(4):2375-2383

[83] Randolph DA, Stephens R, Carruthers CJ, Chaplin DD. Cooperation between Th1 and Th2 cells in a murine model of eosinophilic airway inflammation. The Journal of Clinical Investigation. 1999;**104**(8):1021-1029

[84] Fort MM, Cheung J, Yen D, Li J, Zurawski SM, Lo S, et al. IL-25 induces IL-4, IL-5, and IL-13 and Th2-associated pathologies in vivo. Immunity. 2001;**15**(6):985-995

[85] Fallon PG, Ballantyne SJ, Mangan NE, Barlow JL, Dasvarma A, Hewett DR, et al. Identification of an interleukin (IL)-25-dependent cell population that provides IL-4, IL-5, and IL-13 at the onset of helminth expulsion. The Journal of Experimental Medicine. 2006;**203**(4):1105-1116

[86] Owyang AM, Zaph C, Wilson EH, Guild KJ, McClanahan T, Miller HR, et al. Interleukin 25 regulates type 2 cytokine-dependent immunity and limits chronic inflammation in the gastrointestinal tract. The Journal of Experimental Medicine. 2006;**203**(4):843-849

[87] Wang YH, Angkasekwinai P, Lu N, Voo KS, Arima K, Hanabuchi S, et al. IL-25 augments type 2 immune responses by enhancing the expansion and functions of TSLP-DC-activated Th2 memory cells. The Journal of Experimental Medicine. 2007;**204**(8):1837-1847

[88] Angkasekwinai P, Park H, Wang YH, Wang YH, Chang SH, Corry DB, et al. Interleukin 25 promotes the initiation of proallergic type 2 responses. The Journal of Experimental Medicine. 2007;**204**(7):1509-1517

[89] Ikeda K, Nakajima H, Suzuki K, Kagami S, Hirose K, Suto A, et al. Mast cells produce interleukin-25 upon Fc epsilon RI-mediated activation. Blood. 2003;**101**(9):3594-3596

[90] Dolgachev V, Petersen BC, Budelsky AL, Berlin AA, Lukacs NW. Pulmonary IL-17E (IL-25) production and IL-17RB+ myeloid cell-derived Th2 cytokine production are dependent upon stem cell factor-induced responses during chronic allergic pulmonary disease. Journal of Immunology. 2009;**183**(9):5705-5715

[91] Pan G, French D, Mao W, Maruoka M, Risser P, Lee J, et al. Forced expression of murine IL-17E induces growth retardation, jaundice, a Th2-biased response, and multiorgan inflammation in mice. Journal of Immunology. 2001;**167**(11):6559-6567

[92] de Boer OJ, van der Meer JJ, Teeling P, van der Loos CM, Idu MM, van Maldegem F, et al. Differential expression of interleukin-17 family cytokines in intact and complicated human atherosclerotic plaques. The Journal of Pathology. 2010;**220**(4):499-508

[93] Sonobe Y, Takeuchi H, Kataoka K, Li H, Jin S, Mimuro M, et al. Interleukin-25 expressed by brain

capillary endothelial cells maintains blood-brain barrier function in a protein kinase Cepsilon-dependent manner. The Journal of Biological Chemistry. 2009;**284**(46):31834-31842

[94] Ying S, O'Connor B, Ratoff J, Meng Q, Mallett K, Cousins D, et al. Thymic stromal lymphopoietin expression is increased in asthmatic airways and correlates with expression of Th2-attracting chemokines and disease severity. Journal of Immunology. 2005;**174**(12):8183-8190

[95] West EE, Kashyap M, Leonard WJ. TSLP: A key regulator of asthma pathogenesis. Drug Discovery Today: Disease Mechanisms. 2012;**9**(3-4):83-88

[96] Platts-Mills TAE, de Weck AL, Aalberse RC, Bessot JC, Bjorksten B, Bischoff E, et al. Dust mite allergens and asthma—A worldwide problem. The Journal of Allergy and Clinical Immunology. 1989;**83**(2 Pt 1):416-427

[97] Asosingh K, Weiss K, Queisser K, Wanner N, Yin M, Aronica M, et al. Endothelial cells in the innate response to allergens and initiation of atopic asthma. The Journal of Clinical Investigation. 2018;**128**(7):3116-3128

[98] Belting M, Dorrell MI, Sandgren S, Aguilar E, Ahamed J, Dorfleutner A, et al. Regulation of angiogenesis by tissue factor cytoplasmic domain signaling. Nature Medicine. 2004;**10**(5):502-509

[99] Uusitalo-Jarvinen H, Kurokawa T, Mueller BM, Andrade-Gordon P, Friedlander M, Ruf W. Role of protease activated receptor 1 and 2 signaling in hypoxia-induced angiogenesis. Arteriosclerosis, Thrombosis, and Vascular Biology. 2007;**27**(6):1456-1462

[100] Wara AK, Foo S, Croce K, Sun X, Icli B, Tesmenitsky Y, et al. TGF-beta1 signaling and Kruppel-like factor 10 regulate bone marrow-derived proangiogenic cell differentiation, function, and neovascularization. Blood. 2011;**118**(24):6450-6460

[101] Wara AK, Manica A, Marchini JF, Sun X, Icli B, Tesmenitsky Y, et al. Bone marrow-derived Kruppel-like factor 10 controls reendothelialization in response to arterial injury. Arteriosclerosis, Thrombosis, and Vascular Biology. 2013;**33**(7):1552-1560

[102] Milia AF, Salis MB, Stacca T, Pinna A, Madeddu P, Trevisani M, et al. Protease-activated receptor-2 stimulates angiogenesis and accelerates hemodynamic recovery in a mouse model of hindlimb ischemia. Circulation Research. 2002;**91**(4):346-352

[103] Tomee JF, van Weissenbruch R, de Monchy JG, Kauffman HF. Interactions between inhalant allergen extracts and airway epithelial cells: Effect on cytokine production and cell detachment. The Journal of Allergy and Clinical Immunology. 1998;**102**(1):75-85

[104] Cocks TM, Fong B, Chow JM, Anderson GP, Frauman AG, Goldie RG, et al. A protective role for protease-activated receptors in the airways. Nature. 1999;**398**(6723):156-160

[105] Ricciardolo FL, Steinhoff M, Amadesi S, Guerrini R, Tognetto M, Trevisani M, et al. Presence and bronchomotor activity of protease-activated receptor-2 in guinea pig airways. American Journal of Respiratory and Critical Care Medicine. 2000;**161**(5):1672-1680

[106] Cocks TM, Moffatt JD. Protease-activated receptor-2 (PAR2) in the airways. Pulmonary Pharmacology & Therapeutics. 2001;**14**(3):183-191

[107] Schmidlin F, Amadesi S, Vidil R, Trevisani M, Martinet N, Caughey G,

et al. Expression and function of proteinase-activated receptor 2 in human bronchial smooth muscle. American Journal of Respiratory and Critical Care Medicine. 2001;**164**(7):1276-1281

[108] Pichavant M, Charbonnier AS, Taront S, Brichet A, Wallaert B, Pestel J, et al. Asthmatic bronchial epithelium activated by the proteolytic allergen Der p 1 increases selective dendritic cell recruitment. The Journal of Allergy and Clinical Immunology. 2005;**115**(4):771-778

[109] Adam E, Hansen KK, Astudillo Fernandez O, Coulon L, Bex F, Duhant X, et al. The house dust mite allergen Der p 1, unlike Der p 3, stimulates the expression of interleukin-8 in human airway epithelial cells via a proteinase-activated receptor-2-independent mechanism. The Journal of Biological Chemistry. 2006;**281**(11):6910-6923

[110] Lambrecht BN, Hammad H. The airway epithelium in asthma. Nature Medicine. 2012;**18**(5):684-692

[111] Sun G, Stacey MA, Schmidt M, Mori L, Mattoli S. Interaction of mite allergens Der p3 and Der p9 with protease-activated receptor-2 expressed by lung epithelial cells. Journal of Immunology. 2001;**167**(2):1014-1021

[112] Asokananthan N, Graham PT, Stewart DJ, Bakker AJ, Eidne KA, Thompson PJ, et al. House dust mite allergens induce proinflammatory cytokines from respiratory epithelial cells: The cysteine protease allergen, Der p 1, activates protease-activated receptor (PAR)-2 and inactivates PAR-1. Journal of Immunology. 2002;**169**(8):4572-4578

[113] Willart MA, Deswarte K, Pouliot P, Braun H, Beyaert R, Lambrecht BN, et al. Interleukin-1alpha controls allergic sensitization to inhaled house dust mite via the epithelial release of GM-CSF and IL-33. The Journal of Experimental Medicine. 2012;**209**(8):1505-1517

[114] Stampfli MR, Wiley RE, Neigh GS, Gajewska BU, Lei XF, Snider DP, et al. GM-CSF transgene expression in the airway allows aerosolized ovalbumin to induce allergic sensitization in mice. The Journal of Clinical Investigation. 1998;**102**(9):1704-1714

[115] Ohta K, Yamashita N, Tajima M, Miyasaka T, Nakano J, Nakajima M, et al. Diesel exhaust particulate induces airway hyperresponsiveness in a murine model: Essential role of GM-CSF. Journal of Allergy and Clinical Immunology. 1999;**104**(5):1024-1030

[116] Cates EC, Fattouh R, Wattie J, Inman MD, Goncharova S, Coyle AJ, et al. Intranasal exposure of mice to house dust mite elicits allergic airway inflammation via a GM-CSF-mediated mechanism. Journal of Immunology. 2004;**173**(10):6384-6392

[117] Bleck B, Tse DB, Jaspers I, Curotto de Lafaille MA, Reibman J. Diesel exhaust particle-exposed human bronchial epithelial cells induce dendritic cell maturation. Journal of Immunology. 2006;**176**(12):7431-7437

[118] Zhou Q, Ho AW, Schlitzer A, Tang Y, Wong KH, Wong FH, et al. GM-CSF-licensed CD11b+ lung dendritic cells orchestrate Th2 immunity to Blomia tropicalis. Journal of Immunology. 2014;**193**(2):496-509

[119] Asosingh K, Aldred MA, Vasanji A, Drazba J, Sharp J, Farver C, et al. Circulating angiogenic precursors in idiopathic pulmonary arterial hypertension. The American Journal of Pathology. 2008;**172**(3):615-627

[120] Choo JH, Nagata M, Sutani A, Kikuchi I, Sakamoto Y. Theophylline attenuates the adhesion of eosinophils to endothelial cells. International

Archives of Allergy and Immunology. 2003;**131**(Suppl 1):40-45

[121] Virchow JC Jr, Faehndrich S, Nassenstein C, Bock S, Matthys H, Luttmann W. Effect of a specific cysteinyl leukotriene-receptor 1-antagonist (montelukast) on the transmigration of eosinophils across human umbilical vein endothelial cells. Clinical and Experimental Allergy. 2001;**31**(6):836-844

[122] Takizawa T, Watanabe C, Saiki I, Wada Y, Tohma T, Nagai H. Effects of a new antiallergic drug, VUF-K-8788, on infiltration of lung parenchyma by eosinophils in guinea pigs and eosinophil-adhesion to human umbilical vein endothelial cells (HUVEC). Biological & Pharmaceutical Bulletin. 2001;**24**(10):1127-1132

[123] Hoshino M, Nakamura Y, Hamid QA. Gene expression of vascular endothelial growth factor and its receptors and angiogenesis in bronchial asthma. The Journal of Allergy and Clinical Immunology. 2001;**107**(6):1034-1038

[124] Kanazawa H, Hirata K, Yoshikawa J. Involvement of vascular endothelial growth factor in exercise induced bronchoconstriction in asthmatic patients. Thorax. 2002;**57**(10):885-888

[125] Asai K, Kanazawa H, Otani K, Shiraishi S, Hirata K, Yoshikawa J. Imbalance between vascular endothelial growth factor and endostatin levels in induced sputum from asthmatic subjects. The Journal of Allergy and Clinical Immunology. 2002;**110**(4):571-575

[126] Asai K, Kanazawa H, Kamoi H, Shiraishi S, Hirata K, Yoshikawa J. Increased levels of vascular endothelial growth factor in induced sputum in asthmatic patients. Clinical and Experimental Allergy. 2003;**33**(5):595-599

[127] Papadaki G, Bakakos P, Kostikas K, Hillas G, Tsilogianni Z, Koulouris NG, et al. Vascular endothelial growth factor and cysteinyl leukotrienes in sputum supernatant of patients with asthma. Respiratory Medicine. 2013;**107**(9):1339-1345

[128] Abdel-Rahman AM, el-Sahrigy SA, Bakr SI. A comparative study of two angiogenic factors: Vascular endothelial growth factor and angiogenin in induced sputum from asthmatic children in acute attack. Chest. 2006;**129**(2):266-271

[129] Lee HY, Min KH, Lee SM, Lee JE, Rhee CK. Clinical significance of serum vascular endothelial growth factor in young male asthma patients. The Korean Journal of Internal Medicine. 2017;**32**(2):295-301

Chapter 5

The Role of Platelets in Allergic Inflammation and Asthma

Mirjana Turkalj and Ivana Banic

Abstract

Platelets are a kind of blood cells derived from bone marrow megakaryocytes and play essential roles in thrombosis, hemostasis, and tissue repair. Platelets have been found to be crucially involved in various immune responses and actively involved in the pathogenesis of allergic diseases such as allergic asthma. Patients with allergic asthma have lower platelet counts and increased levels of markers of platelet activation after allergen exposure. Platelets have been found extravascularly in the airways, and platelet products have been measured in bronchoalveolar lavage (BAL) fluid of asthmatic patients. Platelets are also crucially involved in the development of allergic diseases, including the development of allergic asthma via the regulation of allergic inflammation, especially type 2 inflammation mediated by active platelet-derived IL-33 protein activation. Both platelets and IL-33 are activated by tissue damage and involved in biological defense mechanisms and initiation of tissue repair. Therefore, platelets may be involved in the development of steroid-refractory asthma, including irreversible airway remodeling phenotypes.

Keywords: platelets, immune response, asthma, allergic inflammation, IL-33

1. Introduction

Platelets, also known as thrombocytes (from the Greek words *thrombos* meaning clot and *kytos* meaning a vessel, i.e., a cell), are blood components with a well-established role in hemostasis and thrombosis. Platelets are circulating anuclear cell fragments ca. 2 μm in diameter derived from megakaryocytes of the bone marrow, and their production (as well as megakaryocyte production) is regulated by thrombopoietin (also known as megakaryocyte growth and development factor, MGDF). About 10^{11} new platelets are produced daily in a healthy adult individual, and the average life span of circulating platelets is up to 10 days. Platelets respond to vascular injury by clumping and initiation of blood clotting [1]. More specifically, when blood vessels are damaged and bleeding occurs, immediate and appropriate actions are required to prevent excessive blood loss and to repair tissue damage, including injured blood vessels, and platelets play a central role in these processes. The immediate response to vascular injury and bleeding is vasoconstriction, and soon after that, platelets, which normally circulate the bloodstream in a quiescent state due to certain inhibitory signals, adhere and accumulate at the site of vascular endothelium damage. They become activated and release the contents of their granules containing adenosine diphosphate (ADP), thromboxane A2 (TXA2), calcium, platelet-activating factor (PAF), serotonin, etc. This further promotes platelet aggregation and the formation of a temporary and unstable platelet plug

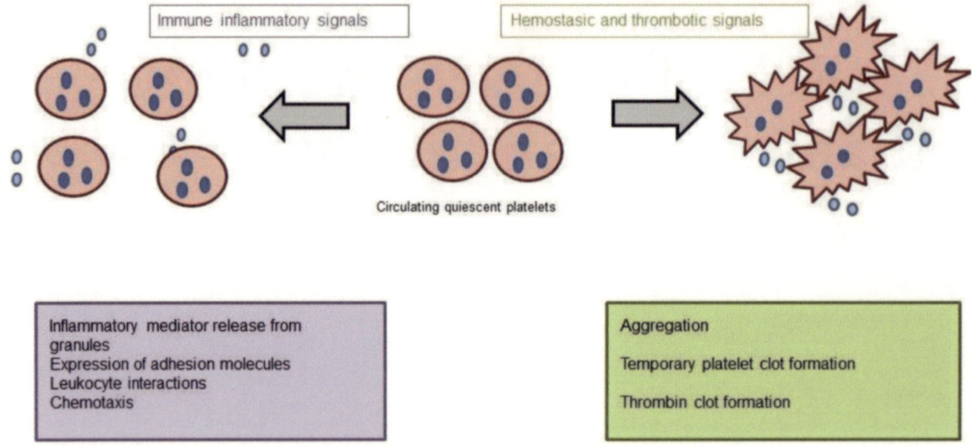

Figure 1.
Dichotomy of platelet functions and activation. Depending on the type of activation signals and mechanisms (prothrombotic or inflammatory), platelets may exhibit either hemostatic and thrombotic (on the right, green box) or proinflammatory effects (on the left, purple box). Red objects indicate platelets (quiescent or activated), while blue objects represent platelet granules.

in a process referred to as primary hemostasis. The activation of a number of coagulation factors leads to the formation of a fibrin mesh which then covers the platelet plug, generating a stable fibrin clot (a process called secondary hemostasis). Logically, once their hemostatic function ceases, clots must be degraded and removed and the tissue damage at the clot site repaired [2, 3]. Undamaged vascular endothelial cells surrounding the clot produce tissue plasminogen activator (tPA) which catalyzes the conversion of plasminogen to active plasmin, a key enzyme involved in clot degradation (fibrinolysis), while the platelets are removed by phagocytosis. Additionally, platelets contain a number of cell and transforming growth factors, including transforming growth factor-β (TGF-β), epidermal growth factor (EGF), and platelet-derived growth factor (PDGF), which play important roles in tissue repair [4].

Since platelets seem to be involved in all processes in response to hemorrhage, including primary and secondary hemostasis, fibrinolysis, and tissue repair, it is conceivable that they may be critical in maintaining the physical barriers to external attacks such as pathogen invasion, including the epithelial barrier integrity and function as well as immune responses, and the body of evidence to support that theory is growing. Indeed, it seems that platelets function quite differently in inflammatory immune responses than they do in hemostasis and thrombosis. Moreover, there are specific and distinct physiological signals and mechanisms in platelet functions involving aggregation (in hemostasis) and those involving immune processes, such as communication and interactions with leukocytes, platelet chemotaxis, as well as direct antimicrobial effects [5]. This has led to the hypothesis of a dichotomy in platelet activation—coagulation vs. their involvement in a plethora of physiologic immune reactions, as well as inflammatory disorders including allergic diseases and asthma [6]. A summary of the dual nature of platelet functions and activation mechanisms is represented in **Figure 1**.

2. Platelet function in the innate and acquired immune responses

Other than posing a risk for serious bleeding, vascular injury represents a significant risk of pathogen invasion. Hence, in addition to a thrombin clot preventing further blood loss, a functional immunological barrier must be formed at the site of vascular damage as soon as possible in order to prevent the spreading of bacteria, viruses, and other pathogens into the body. Platelets exhibit important functions in assisting and directly modulating inflammatory immune responses, which is why they can be considered vital contributors to the integrity of the immunological barrier. These include mechanisms of both the innate and adaptive immunity.

2.1 Immunothrombosis

Tightly regulated and directed thrombosis (called immunothrombosis) in response to vascular injury serves to locally prevent the spread of pathogens to the bloodstream. This process is orchestrated in concordance with platelets and other immune cells, such as neutrophils and monocytes, and initiated either by classical immune cells via their pattern recognition receptors (PRRs) or by the binding of platelets to bacteria. Platelets bind to pathogenic bacteria either directly via thrombocytic pattern recognition receptors to epitopes on bacterial surface or by other plasma proteins that bridge platelets and bacteria [7, 8].

In the process of immunothrombosis, monocytes respond to bacterial pathogen-associated molecular patterns (PAMPs) or damage-associated molecular patterns (DAMPs) by activating extrinsic coagulation pathways with tissue factors (tissue thromboplastin).

Additionally, along with their classical phagocytosis function in response to pathogen invasion, neutrophils facilitate this process by eliminating pathogens by throwing web-like implements or neutrophil extracellular traps (NETs). This process is known as NETosis and represents an alternative type of cell death (other than apoptosis or necrosis). Neutrophils activated in this manner release nuclear DNA and antimicrobial proteins including elastase and myeloperoxidase extracellularly by disrupting their own cell membrane. Pathogens captured by these net-like structures are more easily being phagocytosed. In turn, platelets seem to facilitate NETosis. Platelets are activated, among other stimuli, by binding lipopolysaccharide (LPS) on Gram-negative bacteria via the Toll-like receptor-4 (TLR4). Such activated platelets express P-selectin (or CD62P), a cell adhesion molecule vital in leukocyte recruitment (including neutrophils) to sites of injury via their ligand P-selectin glycoprotein ligand-1 (PSGL-1). This signaling pathway further activates neutrophils to release larger amounts of NETs, and it seems that platelet-neutrophil interactions are essential in the production of NETs since platelet depletion or the disruption of platelet-neutrophil interactions resulted in the proliferation and further diffusion of bacteria in a murine sepsis model. Moreover, NETs also bind tissue factor and activate the intrinsic coagulation pathway by providing its negatively charged surface to the coagulation factor XII and thus participate in immunothrombosis [2, 9–17].

2.2 Platelets are immune cells, de facto

Although they are usually viewed as anuclear cell fragments originating from megakaryocytes involved in hemostasis and thrombosis, platelets exhibit virtually all characteristics of classical immune cells. They contain a number of immune-associated molecules in their intracellular granules, such as P-selectin stored in α-granules in circulating quiescent platelets [18]. When platelets are activated (e.g., by thrombin or ADP), P-selectin is immediately translocated to the plasma membrane [19]. There, it acts as a receptor or ligand for its counterpart expressed on the surface of other immune cells (PSGL-1), such as neutrophils (as described above), monocytes, and lymphocytes, and it is vital for the initiation of the recruitment of these cells to the site of interest [10, 11]. Once activated, platelets secrete a number of other immune-associated molecules, such as chemokines, cytokines, lipid mediators, and growth factors that modulate the inflammatory immune response at the site of vascular injury [4].

Additionally, platelets possess the ability to kill pathogens in both an indirect manner (by recruiting other immune cells) and even directly. Indeed, platelets store a number of molecules with strong antimicrobial potency in their α-granules called platelet microbicidal proteins (PMPs) [20, 21], such as the chemokines CXCL4 (or platelet-factor 4, PF-4) and CXCL-7 (or neutrophil-activating peptide-2, NAP-2) [22, 23]. When activated and bound to bacteria opsonized by immunoglobulin G (IgG), platelets release reactive oxygen species (ROS), antimicrobial peptides, defensins, kinocidins, and proteases, thus killing the pathogen directly [24]. Moreover, other than their involvement in NETosis-mediated pathogen destruction, platelets are involved in other processes directed against microbes involving eosinophil functions similar to NETosis. More specifically, eosinophils and even mast cells are known to produce extracellular DNA traps similar to NETs (called eosinophil extracellular traps, EETs in eosinophils), and certain platelet-derived factors (PAF in combination with IL-5 and GM-CSF) may be involved in the induction and propagation of EETosis [25]. Platelets also express Toll-like receptors 1 through 4 (TLR1-4) and TLR6-9, thus facilitating antigen recognition (PAMPs) and innate immune responses in pathogen destruction [26, 27].

Platelets also express functional receptors of both high and low affinity for immunoglobulins (FcγRI, FcγRII, FcγRIII, FcεRI, FcεRII, FcαRI, etc.) suggesting an important role in adaptive immune response. Moreover, activated platelets express both CD40 and its ligand (CD40L, CD154), which are crucial in antigen presentation to effector cells (T lymphocytes) [28]. Platelet-derived CD40L is also involved in the maturation and activation of dendritic cells (DCs) even extravascularly [29] as well as in the production of T-dependent isotype switching [30].

All of these, along with platelet ability to undergo phagocytosis [31] and chemotaxis to the tissue of interest, emphasize the vital role of platelets in both innate and adaptive immune responses and define them as immune cells de facto. As such, platelets are involved in the pathogenesis of a number of immune disorders, including allergic inflammation and asthma.

3. Role of platelets in allergic inflammation and bronchial asthma

As mentioned before, since platelets may very well be considered immune cells and due to their role in the functioning and integrity of the epithelial and immunological barrier, they are involved in the pathogenesis of a number of chronic diseases, including cancer and inflammatory disorders. Platelet abnormalities in allergy have long been reported, and numerous studies since have underpinned their importance in the regulation of allergic inflammation.

As mentioned before, platelets express both the high- and low-affinity IgE receptors on their surface, and moreover, in allergic donors, exposure to the sensitizing allergen leads to the production of a number of inflammatory mediators, such as serotonin and CCL5 or "regulated on activation, normal T cell expressed and secreted" (RANTES) [32, 33]. In mice with ovalbumin (OVA)-induced allergic inflammation, platelets from ovalbumin-sensitized animals, but not those lacking the high-affinity IgE receptor, migrated extravascularly to the lungs in response to allergic stimuli, thus suggesting that platelets actively participate in antigen-dependent allergic inflammation, including early phases, and via IgE-mediated mechanisms [34].

Additionally, platelets seem to be important for the recruitment of antigen-specific activated T lymphocytes (CD69+ CD4+ T cells) into inflamed airways in patients with allergic asthma. Platelets adhere to the vascular endothelial cells in the airways, and the protein myosin light-chain 9/12 (Myl9/12) in platelets is released to form net-like structures intravascularly. Myl9/12 binds to its ligand on CD69+ T cells and aids their extravasation and migration to the inflamed lungs. In an asthma murine model, blocking of the Myl9/12-CD69 interaction results in reduced airway eosinophilia, indicating that platelets may be crucial for antigen-specific T-cell responses [35].

Exposure to the sensitizing allergen leads to platelet activation in patients with allergic asthma. This allergen challenge may result in a mild peripheral thrombocytopenia (reduced number of platelets), probably due to localized airway recruitment of platelets and the presence of platelet-leukocyte complexes in the blood. Patients with asthma have increased levels of platelet-derived mediators, such as PAF-4, β-thromboglobulin (β-TG), RANTES, and thromboxane, both in the peripheral blood and bronchoalveolar lavage (BAL) fluid, suggesting increased levels of platelet activation. Such platelets are referred to as "exhausted" platelets due to their continuous activation in allergic inflammation, which is why allergic patients may exhibit a mild hemostatic effect associated with shortened platelet survival time and slightly prolonged bleeding time [28]. The role of platelet activation in allergic inflammation reflects also in the fact that an elevated number of platelet precursors (megakaryocytes) has been found in patients who have died of status asthmaticus (an extreme form of asthma exacerbation) [36].

As mentioned before, platelets also produce mitogens, such as TXA2, PDGF, EGF, and vascular endothelial growth factor, which promote airway cell proliferation [37]. Additionally, platelets themselves produce extracellular matrix modifying enzymes and thus participate in airway remodeling characteristic in allergic disorders, such as smooth muscle cell hyperplasia and collagen deposition [5]. Platelet depletion in a murine allergic model resulted in decreased epithelial thickening, smooth muscle thickening, and subepithelial fibrosis [38].

During allergic sensitization, platelets may be activated by the upregulation of their expression of CD154 (CD40L), which plays a central role in mediating the interactions between APCs and lymphocytes. More specifically, platelet-derived CD154 is involved in a number of immune responses, including endothelial cell response, T-helper cell priming, and activation of cytotoxic T lymphocytes. In a murine OVA-induced allergic asthma model, platelet transfer seemed to promote allergic inflammation by enhancing leukocyte infiltration to the affected organ, enhancing the production of IgE, and propagating T-helper type 2 (Th2)-mediated immune responses. On the other hand, platelet depletion in such mice failed to promote asthma development, suggesting that CD154 (CD40L) derived from platelets is required in the progression of allergic asthma. Moreover, platelets seem to inhibit the induction of FoxP3+ regulatory T cells via CD154-mediated mechanisms, which further supports the theory of the vital role of platelet CD154 in allergic disease progression by polarizing Th2-mediated and modifying (inhibiting) Treg-mediated immune responses [39].

In summary, allergic inflammatory stimuli (exposure to a sensitizing allergen) leads to specific platelet activation (other than that in hemostasis, supporting the theory of the dichotomy in platelet functions): the production of a number of inflammatory mediators, such as ROS, RANTES, and 5-hydroxytryptamine (5-HT), a potent spasmogen and bronchoconstrictor, and the generation of platelet-leukocyte complexes resulting in the activation and migration of inflammatory cells to the tissue of interest, thus promoting allergic inflammation and platelet chemotaxis to the affected tissue further propagating the inflammatory immune response. This is schematically represented in **Figure 2**.

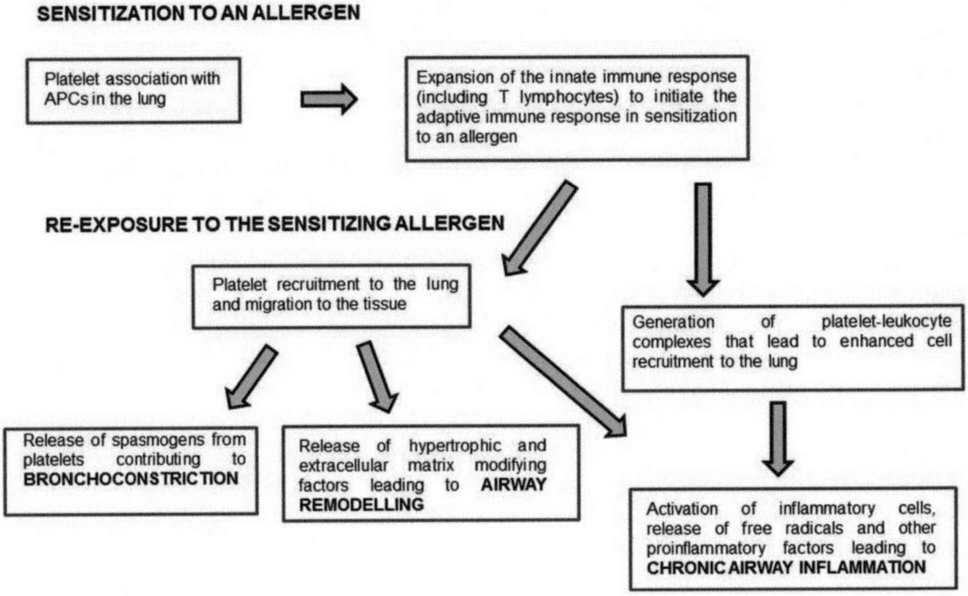

Figure 2.
A summary of the role of platelets in allergic inflammation, more specifically in asthma pathogenesis, in both the sensitization (allergen priming) and subsequent re-exposure phases. APCs, antigen-presenting cells.

4. Role of IL-33 in the immune response

Interleukin-33 (IL-33) is essential in the regulation of innate immune responses, and the body of evidence to underpin its vital role in allergic inflammation and pathogenesis of allergic disorders is growing. IL-33 is a member of the IL-1 superfamily of cytokines that is expressed on a number of cells, including mast cells, DCs, macrophages, fibroblasts, as well as endothelial and epithelial cells. It is a ligand for the interleukin 1 receptor-like 1 (IL1RL1) which is highly expressed on Th2 cells, mast cells, and group 2 innate lymphocytes (ILC2s) [40]. IL-33 exhibits a dual nature in function—it acts as a nuclear factor (binding to DNA) intracellularly and as cytokine extracellularly. As a cytokine, it acts as a potent driver of the production of Th2-cytokines, such as interleukin-4 (IL-4) from Th2 cells, mast cells, eosinophils, and basophils [41, 42].

Genome-wide association studies (GWAS) have identified the *IL33* gene and its receptor (IL1RL1/ST2) as susceptibility loci in allergy and asthma [43, 44].

IL-33 acts as an "alarmin", a factor rapidly released from damaged tissue that serves to alert the immune system of a potential threat of infection. IL-33 is released by necrotic cells after tissue injury and subsequently acts on target cells. In response to IL-33, ILC2s exhibit a strong antigen-non-specific Th2 inflammatory response, suggesting their role in allergy and asthma pathogenesis [2]. ILC2s are activated by IL-33 alone or in combination with IL-2 and subsequently produce large amounts of type 2 cytokines, such as interleukin-5 (IL-5) and interleukin-13 (Il-13) [45]. Intranasal administration of IL-33 to mice significantly induced airway hyperresponsiveness and type 2 inflammation [46]. Moreover, human airway epithelial cells and microvascular endothelial cells in the lung express IL1RL1 and respond to IL-33 stimuli which leads to a rapid production of neutrophil-attracting chemokines [40]. In hemostasis, platelet-derived IL-33 acts on intact tissue cells in proximity of injured blood vessels to produce large amounts of CXCR2 chemokines, thus recruiting neutrophils to the site of injury. Activated platelets further act on neutrophils to release NETs and stimulate neutrophil migration and phagocytosis [2, 40]. Moreover, platelets constitutively express the full length IL-33 and are crucial in the development of papain-induced airway eosinophilia in a murine model via an IL-33-dependent mechanism [47].

IL-33 is also thought to accelerate Th17 cell-mediated airway inflammation via mast cells [48].

5. Platelet-eosinophil interactions in asthma

In asthmatic patients, eosinophilic inflammation is associated with type 2 inflammation; therefore, the interactions between eosinophils and platelets during allergen exposure may be important for the pathogenesis of allergic asthma. In patients with allergic asthma, links in activity between eosinophils and platelets have been found. Levels of ECP and P-selectin as markers of activation of eosinophils and platelets, respectively, were found and suggested a positive association between eosinophils and platelets, which was negatively associated with asthma-related quality of life [49]. Ex *vivo* measurements of eosinophils isolated from patients with asthma have shown that they adhere to endothelial cells more compared to eosinophils from healthy subjects, and platelets seem to promote this adhesion [50]. It is known that the mechanism of interaction between platelets and eosinophils is associated with increased expression of adhesion molecules on activated cells. Expression of P-selectins on platelets was essential for the recruitment of eosinophils into the lung, following allergen challenge [49]. Soluble P-selectins enhanced activation of $\alpha4\beta1$-integrin on eosinophils and stimulate eosinophil adhesion to vascular cell adhesion molecule-1, *in vitro* [51]. After antigen challenge of asthmatic patients, circulating eosinophils associated with P-selectin decreased because of migration of platelet-eosinophil complexes into the lungs [52]. In addition to this mechanism, the interaction between platelets and eosinophils occurs indirectly *via* inflammatory mediator release, such as chemokine PF-4 which is capable of promoting eosinophil-endothelial adhesion due to upregulation of adhesion molecules [53]. The relationship between platelets and eosinophils is synergistic. Eosinophils release cytokines such as platelet-activating factor (PAF) and major basic protein (MBP) which can stimulate and activate platelets [54]. A recent study reported that platelet aggregation was inhibited by the eosinophil cationic protein (ECP) and eosinophil supernatant [55]. The role of eosinophils in platelet aggregation and thrombosis is not yet clear [56]. Certainly there is a therapeutic potential in disrupting eosinophil-platelet interactions in asthmatic patients inhibiting platelet activation and release of platelet cytokines or platelet interaction with other inflammatory cells such as eosinophils. Further research of the interaction between platelets and eosinophils may lead to the design of new therapeutic regimes in allergic asthma [5, 47].

6. Conclusions

Due to the multiplicity of their role in the immune response, platelets can be considered immune cells *de facto*, and there is mounting evidence on their importance in allergic inflammation and asthma pathogenesis. They contribute to all phases of the allergic inflammatory response, including sensitization and subsequent functional and structural changes of the affected tissue, thus perpetuating the chronicity of allergic inflammation. Both platelets and IL-33, an alarmin molecule, are vital in the maintenance and integrity of the immunological barrier.

Moreover, platelets constitutively express IL-33, providing continuous activation signals to target cells, including mast cells and ILCs2, which is crucial in allergic inflammation. Consequently, an emerging therapeutic potential in the inhibition of platelet-dependent inflammation in asthmatic patients may exist.

Conflict of interest

The authors have no conflicts of interest to declare.

Author details

Mirjana Turkalj[1,2,3*] and Ivana Banic[1]

1 Srebrnjak Children's Hospital, Zagreb, Croatia

2 Faculty of Medicine, J.J. Strossmayer University of Osijek, Croatia

3 Catholic University of Croatia, Zagreb, Croatia

*Address all correspondence to: turkalj@bolnica-srebrnjak.hr

References

[1] Laki K. Our ancient heritage in blood clotting and some of its consequences. Annals of the New York Academy of Sciences. 1972;**202**:297-307. DOI: 10.1111/j.1749-6632.1972.tb16342.x

[2] Takeda T, Morita H, Saito H, Matsumoto K. Recent advances in understanding the roles of blood platelets in the pathogenesis of allergic inflammation and bronchial asthma. Allergology International. 2018;**67**: 326-333. DOI: 10.1016/j.alit.2017.11.008

[3] Brass LF. Thrombin and platelet activation. Chest. 2003;**124**:18S-25S. DOI: 10.1378/chest.124.3_suppl.18S

[4] Semple JW, Italiano JE Jr, Freedman J. Platelets and the immune continuum. Nature Reviews. Immunology. 2011;**11**:264-274. DOI: 10.1038/nri2956

[5] Shah SA, Page CP, Pitchford SC. Platelet-eosinophil interactions as a potential therapeutic target in allergic inflammation and asthma. Frontiers in Medicine. 2017;**4**:129. DOI: 10.3389/fmed.2017.00129

[6] Page CP. The involvement of platelets in non-thrombotic processes. Trends in Pharmacological Sciences. 1987;**9**:66-71. DOI: 10.1016/0165-6147(88)90120-4

[7] Jenne CN, Urrutia R, Kubes P. Platelets: Bridging hemostasis, inflammation, and immunity. International Journal of Laboratory Hematology. 2013;**35**:254-261. DOI: 10.1111/ijlh.12084

[8] Cox D, Kerrigan SW, Watson SP. Platelets and the innate immune system: Mechanisms of bacterial-induced platelet activation. Journal of Thrombosis and Haemostasis. 2011;**9**:1097-1107. DOI: 10.1111/j.1538-7836.2011.04264.x

[9] Gaertner F, Massberg S. Blood coagulation in immunothrombosis–At the frontline of intravascular immunity. Seminars in Immunology. 2016;**28**: 561-569. DOI: 10.1016/j.smim.2016.10.010

[10] Larsen E, Celi A, Gilbert GE, Furie BC, Erban JK, Bonfanti R, et al. PADGEM protein: A receptor that mediates the interaction of activated platelets with neutrophils and monocytes. Cell. 1989;**59**:305-312

[11] Diacovo TG, Puri KD, Warnock RA, Springer TA, von Andrian UH. Platelet-mediated lymphocyte delivery to high endothelial venules. Science. 1996;**273**:252-255

[12] Brinkmann V, Reichard U, Goosmann C, Fauler B, Uhlemann Y, Weiss DS, et al. Neutrophil extracellular traps kill bacteria. Science. 2004;**303**:1532-1535. DOI: 10.1126/science.1092385

[13] McDonald B, Urrutia R, Yipp BG, Jenne CN, Kubes P. Intravascular neutrophil extracellular traps capture bacteria from the bloodstream during sepsis. Cell Host & Microbe. 2012;**12**:324-333. DOI: 10.1016/j.chom.2012.06.011

[14] Yipp BG, Kubes P. NETosis: How vital is it? Blood. 2013;**122**:2784-2794. DOI: 10.1182/blood-2013-04-457671

[15] Parker H, Albrett AM, Kettle AJ, Winterbourn CC. Myeloperoxidase associated with neutrophil extracellular traps is active and mediates bacterial killing in the presence of hydrogen peroxide. Journal of Leukocyte Biology. 2012;**91**:369-376. DOI: 10.1189/jlb.0711387

[16] Clark SR, Ma AC, Tavener SA, McDonald B, Goodarzi Z, Kelly MM, et al. Platelet TLR4 activates neutrophil extracellular traps to ensnare bacteria in septic blood. Nature Medicine. 2007;**13**:463-469. DOI: 10.1038/nm1565

[17] Sreeramkumar V, Adrover JM, Ballesteros I, Cuartero MI, Rossaint J, Bilbao I, et al. Neutrophils scan for activated platelets to initiate inflammation. Science. 2014;**346**: 1234-1238. DOI: 10.1126/science.1256478

[18] Stenberg PE, McEver RP, Shuman MA, Jacques YV, Bainton DF. A platelet alpha-granule membrane protein (GMP-140) is expressed on the plasma membrane after activation. The Journal of Cell Biology. 1985;**101**:890-896

[19] Johnston GI, Cook RG, McEver RP. Cloning of GMP-140, a granule membrane protein of platelets and endothelium: Sequence similarity to proteins involved in cell adhesion and inflammation. Cell. 1989;**56**:1033-1044

[20] Yeaman MR. Platelets: At the nexus of antimicrobial defence. Nature Reviews. Microbiology. 2104;**12**: 426-437. DOI: 10.1038/nrmicro3269

[21] Yeaman MR, Norman DC, Bayer AS. Platelet microbicidal protein enhances antibiotic-induced killing and postantibiotic effect in Staphylococcus aureus. Antimicrobial Agents and Chemotherapy. 1992;**36**:1665-1670

[22] Yeaman MR, Yount NY, Waring AJ, Gank KD, Kupferwasser D, Wiese R, et al. Modular determinants of antimicrobial activity in platelet factor-4 family kinocidins. Biochimica et Biophysica Acta. 2007;**1768**:609-619. DOI: 10.1016/j.bbamem.2006.11.010

[23] Krijgsveld J, Zaat SA, Meeldijk J, van Veelen PA, Fang G, Poolman B, et al. Thrombocidins, microbicidal proteins from human blood platelets, are C-terminal deletion products of CXC chemokines. The Journal of Biological Chemistry. 2000;**275**:20374-20381. DOI: 10.1074/jbc.275.27.20374

[24] Palankar R, Kohler TP, Krauel K, Wesche J, Hammerschmidt S, Greinacher A. Platelets kill bacteria by bridging innate and adaptive immunity via platelet factor 4 and FcγRIIA. Journal of Thrombosis and Haemostasis. 2018;**16**:1187-1197. DOI: 10.1111/jth.13955

[25] Ueki S, Melo RC, Ghiran I, Spencer LA, Dvorak AM, Weller PF. Eosinophil extracellular trap cell death mediates lytic release of free secretion-competent eosinophil granules in humans. Blood. 2013;**121**:2074-2083. DOI: 10.1182/blood-2012-05-432088

[26] Hamzeh-Cognasse H, Damien P, Chabert A, Pozzetto B, Cognasse F, Garraud O. Platelets and infections-complex interations with bacteria. Frontiers in Immunology. 2015;**6**:82. DOI: 10.3389/fimmu.2015.00082

[27] Cognasse F, Nguyen KA, Damien P, McNicol A, Pozzetto B, Hamzeh-Cognasse H, et al. The inflammatory role of platelets via their TLRs and Siglec receptors. Frontiers in Immunology. 2015;**6**:83. DOI: 10.3389/fimmu.2015.00083

[28] Idzko M, Pitchford S, Page C. Role of platelets in allergic airway inflammation. The Journal of Allergy and Clinical Immunology. 2015;**135**:1416-1423. DOI: 10.1016/j.jaci.2015.04.028

[29] Durk T, Duerschmied D, Muller T, Grimm M, Reuter S, Vieira RP, et al. Production of serotonin by tryptophan hydroxylase 1 and release via platelets contribute to allergic airway inflammation. American Journal of Respiratory and Critical Care Medicine. 2013;**187**:476-485. DOI: 10.1164/rccm.201208-1440OC

[30] Elzey BD, Ratliff TL, Sowa JM, Crist SA. Platelet CD40L at the interface of adaptive immunity. Thrombosis Research. 2011;**127**:180-183. DOI: 10.1016/j.thromres.2010.10.011

[31] Youssefian T, Drouin A, Masse JM, Guichard J, Cramer EM. Host defense

role of platelets: Engulfment of HIV and Staphylococcus aureus occurs in a specific subcellular compartment and is enhanced by platelet activation. Blood. 2002;**99**:4021-4029. DOI: 10.1182/blood-2001-12-0191

[32] Joseph M, Gounni AS, Kusnierz JP, Vorng H, Sarfati M, Kinet JP, et al. Expression and functions of the high-affinity IgE receptor on human platelets and megakaryocyte precursors. European Journal of Immunology. 1997;**27**:2212-2218. DOI: 10.1002/eji.1830270914

[33] Hasegawa S, Tashiro N, Matsubara T, Furukawa S, Ra C. A comparison of FCepsilonRI-mediated RANTES release from human platelets between allergic patients and healthy individuals. International Archives of Allergy and Immunology. 2001;**125**:42-47. DOI: 10.1159/000053852

[34] Pitchford SC, Momi S, Baglioni S, Casali L, Giannini S, Rossi R, et al. Allergen induces the migration of platelets to lung tissue in allergic asthma. American Journal of Respiratory and Critical Care Medicine. 2008;**177**:604-612. DOI: 10.1164/rccm.200702-214OC

[35] Hayashizaki K, Kimura MY, Tokoyoda K, Hosokawa H, Shinoda K, Hirahara K, et al. Myosin light chains 9 and 12 are functional ligands for CD69 that regulate allergic inflammation. Science Immunology. 2016;**1**:eaaf9154. DOI: 10.1126/sciimmunol.aaf9154

[36] Slater D, Martin J, Trowbridge A. The platelet in asthma. Lancet. 1985;**1**:110

[37] Page C, Pitchford S. Platelets and allergic inflammation. Clinical & Experimental Allergy. 2014;**44**:90-913. DOI: 10.1111/cea.12322

[38] Pitchford SC, Riffo-Vasquez Y, Sousa A, Momi S, Gressele P, Spina D, et al. Platelets are necessary for airway wall remodeling in a murine model of chronic allergic inflammation. Blood. 2004;**103**:639-647. DOI: 10.1182/blood-2003-05-1707

[39] Tian J, Zhu T, Liu J, Guo Z, Cao X. Platelets promote allergic asthma through the expression of CD154. Cellular & Molecular Immunology. 2015;**12**:700-707. DOI: 10.1038/cmi.2014.111

[40] Yagami A, Orihara K, Morita H, Futamura K, Hashimoto N, Matsumoto K, et al. IL-33 mediates inflammatory responses in human lung tissue cells. Journal of Immunology. 2010;**185**:5743-5750. DOI: 10.4049/jimmunol.0903818

[41] Mirchandani AS, Salmond RJ, Liew FY. Interleukin-33 and the function of innate lymphoid cells. Trends in Immunology. 2012;**33**:389-396. DOI: 10.1016/j.it.2012.04.005

[42] Baekkevold ES, Roussigné M, Yamanaka T, Johansen FE, Jahnsen FL, Amalric F, et al. Molecular characterization of NF-HEV, a nuclear factor preferentially expressed in human high endothelial venules. The American Journal of Pathology. 2003;**163**:69-79. DOI: 10.1016/S0002-9440(10)63631-0

[43] Moffatt MF, Gut IG, Demenais F, Strachan DP, Bouzigon E, Heath S, et al. A large-scale, consortium-based genomewide association study of asthma. The New England Journal of Medicine. 2010;**363**:1211-1221. DOI: 10.1056/NEJMoa0906312

[44] Hinds DA, McMahon G, Kiefer AK, Do CB, Eriksson N, Evans DM, et al. A genome-wide association meta-analysis of self-reported allergy identifies shared and allergy-specific susceptibility loci. Nature Genetics. 2013;**45**:907-911. DOI: 10.1038/ng.2686

[45] Neil DR, Wong SH, Bellosi A, Flynn RJ, Daly M, Langford TK, et al.

Noucytes represent a new innate effector leukocyte that mediates type-2 immunity. Nature. 2010;**464**:1367-1370. DOI: 10.1038/nature08900

[46] Kondo Y, Yoshimoto T, Yasuda K, Futatsugi-Yumikura S, Morimoto M, Hayashi N, et al. Administration of IL-33 induces airway hyperresponsiveness and goblet cell hyperplasia in the lungs in the absence of adaptive immune system. International Immunology. 2008;**20**: 791-800. DOI: 10.1093/intimm/dxn037

[47] Takeda T, Unno H, Morita H, Futamura K, Emi-Sugie M, Arae K, et al. Platelets constitutively express IL-33 protein and modulate eosinophilic airway inflammation. Journal of Allergy and Clinical Immunology. 2016;**138**:1395-1403. DOI: 10.1016/j.jaci.2016.01.032

[48] Cho KA, Suh JW, Sohn JH, Park JW, Lee H, Kang JL, et al. IL-33 induces Th17-mediated airway inflammation via mast cells in ovalbumin-challenged mice. American Journal of Physiology. Lung Cellular and Molecular Physiology. 2012;**302**:L429-L440. DOI: 10.1152/ajplung.00252.2011

[49] Benton AS, Kumar N, Lerner J, Wiles AA, Foerster M, Teach SJ, et al. Airway platelet activation is associated with airway eosinophilic inflammation in asthma. Journal of Investigative Medicine. 2010;**58**:987. DOI: 10.231/JIM.0b013e3181fa02f7

[50] Ulfman LH, Joosten DP, van Aalst CW, Lammers JW, van de Graaf EA, Koenderman L, et al. Platelets promote eosinophil adhesion of patients with asthma to endothelium under flow conditions. American Journal of Respiratory Cell and Molecular Biology. 2003;**28**:512-519. DOI: 10.1165/rcmb.4806

[51] Johansson MW, Mosher DF. Activation of β1 integrins on blood eosinophils by P-selectin. American Journal of Respiratory Cell and Molecular Biology. 2011;**45**:889-997. DOI: 10.1165/rcmb.2010-0402OC

[52] Johansson MW, Han ST, Gunderson KA, Busse WW, Jarjour NN, Mosher DF. Platelet activation, P-selectin, and eosinophil β1-integrin activation in asthma. American Journal of Respiratory and Critical Care Medicine. 2012;**185**:498-507. DOI: 10.1164/rccm.201109-1712OC

[53] Zuchtriegel G, Uhl B, Puhr-Westerheide D, Pörnbacher M, Lauber K, Krombach F, et al. Platelets guide leukocytes to their sites of extravasation. PLoS Biology. 2016;**14**:e1002459. DOI: 10.1371/journal.pbio.1002459

[54] Rohrbach MS, Wheatley CL, Slifman NR, Gleich GJ. Activation of platelets by eosinophil granule proteins. The Journal of Experimental Medicine. 1990;**172**:1271-1274

[55] Maziero AM, Lorenzetti R, Donato JL, Lilla S, De Nucci G. Inhibition of human platelet aggregation by eosinophils. Life Sciences. 2013;**93**: 416-422. DOI: 10.1016/j.lfs.2013.07.012

[56] Kanabar V, Tedaldi L, Jiang J, Nie X, Panina I, Descroix K, et al. Base-modified UDP-sugars reduce cell surface levels of P-selectin glycoprotein 1 (PSGL-1) on IL-1β-stimulated human monocytes. Glycobiology. 2016;**26**: 1059-1071. DOI: 10.1093/glycob/cww053

Chapter 6

Eosinophilic Asthma

Bushra Mubarak, Huma Shakoor and Fozia Masood

Abstract

Eosinophilic asthma is known as a main phenotype of asthma classified on the basis of immune cells involved in inflammatory response in the respiratory airway. Eosinophilic asthma can be related to increased severity of asthma, allergic sensitization, adult onset, and increased resistance to corticosteroids. The prevalence of eosinophilic asthma is 32–40% among asthmatic patients. Different cells and cytokines are involved in its pathogenesis including eosinophil, mast cells, type 2 helper T cells, innate lymphoid cells, IL-4, IL-5, and IL-13. Eosinophil count in induced sputum and bronchoalveolar lavage is the yardstick for recognizing and distinguishing eosinophilic asthma from non-eosinophilic asthma, while various tests which are noninvasive such as fractional exhaled nitric oxide and periostin are arising as possible substitutes. Novel and advanced therapies new and advanced therapies and more convenient biological drugs, Leads to high requirement for particular endotype- and phenotype-related treatment plans. Identification and knowledge of the specific pathophysiology of eosinophilic asthma have great association with disease management and chances for better patient prognosis.

Keywords: eosinophilic asthma, phenotype, mast cells, Th2 cell, ILCs, interleukin-5

1. Introduction

Asthma is a Greek word which means "labored breathing." Asthma is a common disease which is characterized by reversible airway inflammation, chronic airway blockage, hyperresponsiveness, wheezing, and cough arising spontaneously and in reaction to nonspecific environmental factors. It affects an approximately 358 million people worldwide, causing a significant burden on healthcare systems. The highest prevalence of asthma has been found in the United Kingdom (15%) followed by Australia (14.7%), Canada (14.1%), and the United States (10.9%). In Asia the highest incidence of asthma has been recorded in Japan (6.7%), followed by Iran (5.5%), Pakistan (4.3%), Bangladesh (3.8%), and India (3%) and lowest in China (2.1%) [1]. It is a complex multifactorial disorder with various predisposing factors in environment and genes in which genetics of the individual plays a vital role [2]. Genome-wide studies have reported different loci that are associated with asthma. Asthma is associated directly with genes such as heterogeneity in Fc epsilon receptor 1 (FcεR1) on 11th and q region of 5th chromosome 11, while some other gene polymorphisms have no direct link with asthma.

Asthma usually starts in infancy or young age. Wheezing in early childhood does not always lead to asthma in late childhood. As a matter of fact, wheezing in infancy is commonly related to those children whose airways are relatively small than normal children. They will likely wheeze when they have viral bronchitis. On the other hand, pulmonary function starts off at normal range in children who frequently progress to asthma. After asthma development, their lungs will not develop due to continuous inflammation of their disease.

After genetics, another factor is the environment in which atopy is the most critical cause of asthma. Most of the asthmatic persons have had skin allergy in childhood followed by nasal allergy which leads to asthma. This series of events is called allergic march. Other factors in environment such as construction designs of houses, pollution, dust mites, molds, pet denders, particles of cockroach waste, tobacco smoke, inhalation of cold and dry air, food and infection are trigger factors to cause asthma. Today, our residence and daily activities have changed such as homes are more heated as well as isolated. Taking a bath and showers more frequently leads to more moisture inside the homes. These changes have made our house environment friendlier for house dust mites. Diet has also changed such as seasonal fruits and vegetables switched to artificially ripened fruits. This simulated ripening of fruits may alter their chemical structure and antigenicity [3]. Air pollutants that have been rising due to vehicular traffic are ozone, particulates, and nitrogen oxide. Air pollutant affects asthma by increasing IgE production, imposing oxidative stress on airways directly and indirectly, functioning as a vector for allergens, and enhancing release of IL-4 and histamine from basophils [4] (**Figure 1**).

There is a close relationship between infections and asthma exacerbation. Increased exposure to infection of respiratory viruses is protective against asthma development. This is called hygiene hypothesis. Different researches on children revealed protective effect of infections in farming communities. Infants who drink unpasteurized milk or are taken to the animal house have a reduced chance of allergy and asthma, but there is no protective effect of infections if children are exposed only after 1 year of age. Once asthma is developed, viral diseases can

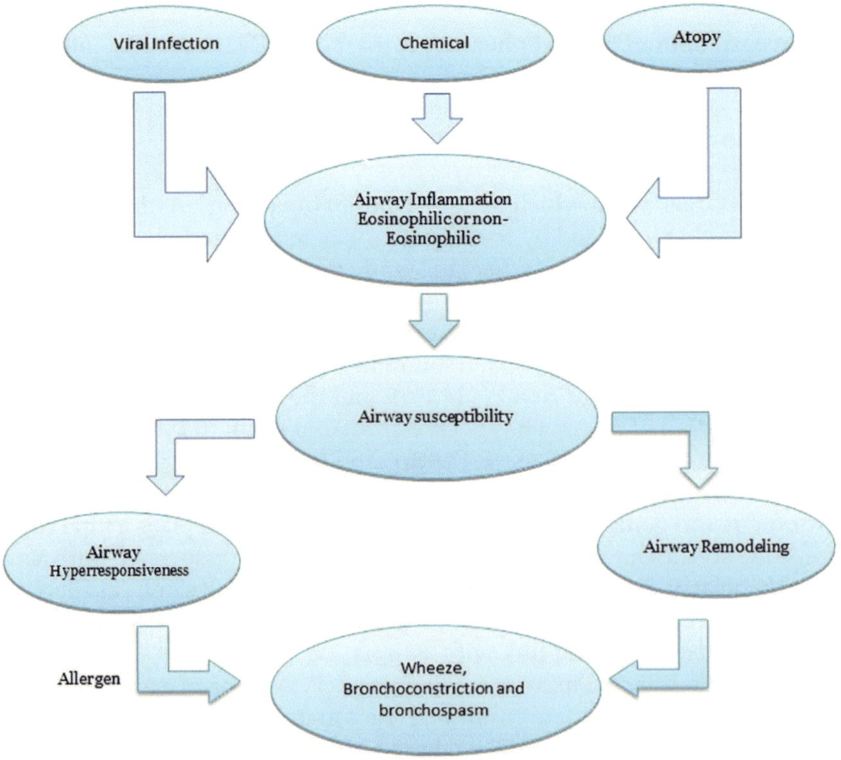

Figure 1.
The role of atopy and other environmental factors in asthma.

exacerbate its symptoms because viruses increase airway inflammation linked with asthma. Bacterial and parasitic infections can minimize the risk of allergy by reducing IgE sensitization and weakening the airways' response to allergen [5].

1.1 Classification of asthma

Asthma is a complex heterogeneous disease with variety of phenotypes. A disease phenotype gives information about clinical and morphological characteristics of disease, triggers, and therapy response but does not describe about pathogenesis of disease. Due to this reason, the classification of asthma has been further clarified with the development of endotypes, which is based on pathological mechanisms and treatment responses of asthma.

There is an overlap in this classification. Each endotype of asthma can have several phenotypes, just as a specific phenotype may be linked with more than one endotype [6]. These phenotypes have distinct subtypes based on symptoms, triggers, age at onset of disease, severity of disease, and underlying inflammation. Traditionally, asthma has been classified into extrinsic/atopic and intrinsic/nonatopic asthma. Atopic asthma starts in children who have family members with history of allergy and good treatment response. Atopic asthma usually begins after allergen exposure. On the other hand, intrinsic asthma is developed in adult age, and family history is absent in this type of asthma. Intrinsic asthma is a nonallergic type of asthma caused by cold, humidity, strong smells, infections (viral-induced asthma), and chemicals in smoke and cigarette. Nonallergic asthma occurs in 10–33% of asthmatic patients [7].

Asthma can also be divided into early-onset and late-onset asthma according to age of presentation of disease. Symptom-based asthma includes chronic asthma, acute severe asthma, brittle asthma, nocturnal asthma, and exercise-induced asthma. On the basis of frequency and severity of symptoms, the Global Initiative for Asthma (GINA) has classified asthma into intermittent, mild persistent, moderated persistent, and severe persistent asthma [8]. The American Thoracic Society and European Respiratory Society have also classified asthma into refractory asthma and "difficult/therapy-resistant asthma" based on the medication plan to achieve good control on asthma [9]. The World Health Organization (WHO) divided severe asthma into untreated severe asthma, difficult-to-treat asthma, and treatment-resistant severe asthma [10]. Based on etiology and underlying inflammation, asthma has also been classified into eosinophilic and non-eosinophilic (neutrophilic and paucigranulocytic) asthma [11].

1.2 Eosinophilic asthma

Eosinophilic asthma is a specific phenotype of asthma that is defined by inflammation of the basement membrane in the airway mucosa and high eosinophil levels in sputum and blood compared with non-eosinophilic asthma where no typical thickening of the basement membrane has been seen. Repeated asthma exacerbations are more noticeable in patients of eosinophilic than non-eosinophilic asthma [12]. Even though the exact incidence of eosinophilic asthma is not known, among patients with severe asthma who show about 5–10% of the asthmatic people, sputum eosinophilia (≥2%) or blood (≥300 cells/μl) can be observed in 32–40% of population which are linked with recurrent asthma exacerbations, as well as disease severity [13]. A subgroup of patients of eosinophilic asthma maintains constant airways and sputum eosinophilia even with conventional corticosteroid therapy called steroid-resistant eosinophilic asthma. In different studies, the levels of eosinophil in sputum are high in asthmatics with severe disease [14].

Eosinophilic asthma has three distinct presentations. The first phenotype of eosinophilic asthma is termed as allergen-exacerbated asthma in whom patients show allergen sensitization (atopy), accompanied with allergic rhinitis, present with exacerbated symptoms on allergen exposure and common in early-onset asthma [7, 15]. The second phenotype of eosinophilic asthma comprises those individuals in whom the eosinophilic inflammation is a prominent pathology, but these patients are nonatopic and can present at any age especially in adult age. This phenotype is called idiopathic eosinophilic asthma [7, 16]. Aspirin-exacerbated respiratory disease is the third phenotype of eosinophilic asthma with distinct features comprised of the presence of severe rhinosinusitis with nasal polyps and aspirin sensitivity. Like idiopathic eosinophilic asthma, aspirin-exacerbated respiratory disease is also presented in adulthood and nonatopic patients. However, different studies have documented that a small number of patients who developed asthma early in life showed 36% tissue eosinophilia, in comparison with the late-onset asthma which had 63% eosinophil level [17].

2. Pathophysiological mechanism

Asthma is a complex disease characterized by different pathological mechanisms including inflammation, hyperresponsiveness, remodeling, and angiogenesis of airways (**Figure 2**).

2.1 Airway inflammation

Eosinophilic airway inflammation is the main pathophysiological mechanism of eosinophilic asthma. Eosinophilic asthma develops from complex immunologic and pro-inflammatory mechanisms, mainly driven by T helper 2 (Th2) cells, which is a part of adaptive immunity release interleukins (IL-5, IL-4, and IL-13). Besides being orchestrated by mechanisms of adaptive immunity, Th2-mediated airway eosinophilia can be also linked with innate immunity, which relied on intercellular connection comprising of dendritic cells, bronchial epithelial cells, and innate lymphoid cells. As a result, airway eosinophilia arises due to the biological activity of both type 2 helper T (Th2) and type 2 innate lymphoid (ILC2) cells, which are critically participating in the pathogenic process of type-2 inflammation in eosinophilic allergic and nonallergic asthma [18]. These mechanisms are linked with increased IgE expression. In eosinophilic asthma patients, eosinophils collect in the respiratory tract. Differentiation of Th2 lymphocytes needs the association of various promoting elements, including costimulatory molecules and interleukins released by dendritic cells and inflammatory cells.

Eosinophilic allergic asthma is caused by aeroallergen like pollen and house dust mite which have proteolytic characteristics and also have small amount of bacterial components like lipopolysaccharides (LPS) [19]. Thus, on entrance into the respiratory epithelial membrane, allergens can attach with the Toll-like receptor (TLR), a receptor which is involved in innate immunity. Upon TLR activation, epithelial cells produce cytokines including thymic stromal lymphopoietin (TSLP), IL-25, and IL-33 which are capable of developing adaptive immune response of Th2 type. Moreover, TLR activation also evokes the secretion of chemokines such as CCL2 and CCL20, which increase the maturation of dendritic cells [20]. These dendritic cells move into the lumen of airways, take aeroallergens, and break them in the cytoplasm, leading to the generation of peptide fragments of allergen. These fragments are presented by class II HLA molecules on dendritic cells that move to regional lymph nodes where these antigen fragments are presented to T lymphocytes [21].

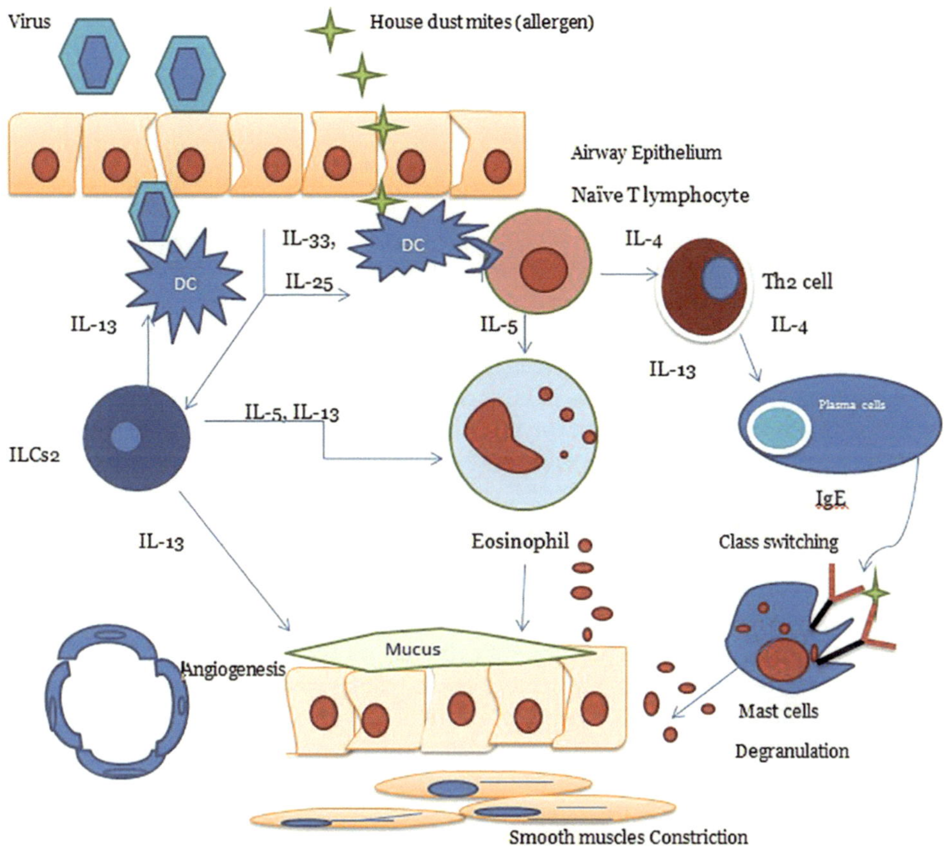

Figure 2.
Pathogenesis of eosinophilic asthma. Asthma arises from interaction between genetic and environmental factors including allergens and viruses. Allergens or viruses can be caught by dendritic cells (DCs) located in the epithelium, which process and present antigen to naive (Th0) T helper cells. This allergen activates Th0 to Th2 cells which produce IL-4 and IL-13. These cytokines activate B cell for class switching to IgE immunoglobulin. Further, Th2 cells also secrete IL-5, which activates and recruits eosinophil. IgE-dependent degranulation of mast cells secretes both immediate and newly formed mediators like leukotriene, prostaglandin cytokines, etc. other important cells contributing to asthma pathobiology are type 2 innate lymphoid cell (ILCs2), producing IL-13 and IL-5 which cause eosinophil recruitment and expansion in nonallergic eosinophilic asthma.

After activation of T-cell receptors by antigenic peptides, sensitization and stimulation of adaptive immune system take place. Stimulation of naive T lymphocytes needs the attachment of their costimulatory molecules (CD28, ICOS, and OX40) with their ligand present on dendritic cells (CD80/B7.1, CD86/B7.2, ICOS ligand, and OX40 ligand). Differentiation of T lymphocytes is critically dependent on the cytokine environment [22]. Th2 polarization requires high levels of IL-4 and low concentration of IL-12. IL-4 is secreted by mast cells and basophils. GATA3 is the main transcription factor present in type 2 helper T cells that promote the production of Th2-type cytokines including IL-4, IL-5, IL-9, and IL-13. These interleukins cause eosinophils and mast cells' maturation and recruitment, promoting immunoglobulin class switching to IgE production. As a result, cytotoxic products released by degranulation of eosinophils induce airway epithelial injury, mucus hyperproduction, bronchial hyperresponsiveness, impaired ciliary movement, and an increase in smooth muscle size [23].

The late-onset type of eosinophilic asthma that is usually nonallergic arises in the absence of stimulation of Th2 lymphocytes. Recent researches suggest that the main role in the development of eosinophilic nonallergic asthma is played by

ILC2s which is activated by IL-25, by IL-33, and by prostaglandin D2 (PGD2) [24]. Consequently, these two distinct pro-inflammatory routes driven by either Th2 lymphocytes or innate ILC2s produce IL-5 which is mainly involved in eosinophilic inflammation of airways in asthma.

2.2 Airway hyperresponsiveness

Chronic inflammation of airways in asthma leads to more rapid contraction of smooth muscles of airways than in normal person in effect of broad range of stimuli, a condition termed airway hyperresponsiveness [25]. Airway hyperresponsiveness is a result of eosinophil infiltration mediated by T lymphocyte-secreted factor called eosinophil chemotactic factor (ECF-L). Hyper responsiveness of the air ways is caused by the decrease in function of neuronal M2 muscarinic receptor on parasympathetic nerves in the lungs due to eosinophil's major basic protein which is a protein released from granules of eosinophils. Schwartz et al. reported a direct relationship between eosinophil count in the airways, sputum and peripheral blood, and airway hyperresponsiveness [26].

2.3 Airway remodeling

Airway remodeling is the permanent cellular and structural modification in the airways primarily due to repair mechanisms in reaction to chronic inflammation. In a broad term, the airway is modified so that it acts in a different manner when allergens or nonspecific factors like exercise, cold air, perfume, and smoke are induced into the patient and it leads to irreversible change of lung functions [27]. There are various changes in structural and physiological characteristics which are different in every asthmatic patient. Most noticeable structural change is thickening of basement membrane of airway which is due to accumulation of type III collagen produced by myofibroblast. These myofibroblastic cells are stimulated and controlled by growth factors secreted by the epithelial cells and various cytokines (transforming growth factor-β (TGF-β), IL-10, and IL-17) released by T lymphocytes and eosinophils that have profibrotic responses while at the same time down-regulating the function of T and B lymphocytes [28].

Previously, it was thought that the airways' epithelial membrane is an innocent sufferer, becoming injured and lost due to the effect of toxic agents secreted by eosinophils and other inflammatory cells. But now, it has been reported that growth factors and interleukins (IL-8) secreted by the cells of epithelial membrane perform an active role in remodeling. Metalloproteases and epidermal growth factors released from matrix on inflammation stimulate these chemokines. On chemokine activation, neutrophils and other immune cells attracted to the area of damage cause structural alterations in the airways. Other structural changes including mucus metaplasia and increased angiogenesis have also been observed in asthmatic patients [29].

2.4 Angiogenesis

There is a rise in the number of blood arteries in the medium and small respiratory airway submucosa. It may help in physiological changes in airways of patients with asthma, including asthma due to exercise. Several studies have been documented that vascular endothelial growth factor (VEGF) may contribute in angiogenesis. High expression of VEGF has been observed due to hypoxia and several cytokines and growth factors such as epidermal growth factor, TGF-β, IL-1α, and IL-6. VEGF expression is decreased by other interleukins including IL-10 and IL-13 [30].

2.5 Role of eosinophil in pathogenesis

Eosinophils are granulocytes in blood produced in the bone marrow with other white blood cells making about 1–3% of white blood cells. Eosinophil plays multiple functions and is an important component of allergic and asthmatic type 2 immune responses. Allergens on exposure starts a group of processes by Th2 cytokine-producing cells, resulting in eosinophils' attraction to the airway through the action of IL-5, and eotaxin research reported that Clara cells of the airway epithelium are the main source of eotaxin in the lung [30].

During asthma attack, eosinophils are stimulated to release proteins from granules including major basic protein, eosinophil peroxidase, eosinophil cationic protein, and eosinophil-derived neurotoxin, all of which are toxic to the epithelial cells of airway. Furthermore, eosinophils secrete plenty of inflammatory mediators like cytokines (interleukins IL-13 and IL-5), platelet-activating factor, growth factors (TGF-α and TGF-β), leukotrienes, thromboxane, and prostaglandins. The secretion of all these mediators results in enhancement of the inflammatory process, airways' epithelium cell injury, airway hyperresponsiveness, mucus hypersecretion, and airway remodeling and bronchospasm [31]. Eosinophils control the allergen-dependent Th2 pulmonary immune responses activated by dendritic cells and T cells as well as decrease Th1 responses [32].

2.6 Role of IL-5 in pathogenesis

Although various bioactive proteins such as IL-3 and granulocyte-macrophage colony-stimulating factor affect the life cycle of eosinophils, eosinophils react mainly to IL-5. Th2 cells, ILCs2, mast cells, natural killer T (NKT) cells, and eosinophils produce IL-5 within respiratory air passage of sufferer with eosinophilic asthma. In asthmatic patients, the bone marrow responds to environmental irritant by rising eosinophil production, and in asthmatics presenting both acute and late asthmatic reactions, this event is related with increased IL-5 mRNA proportion than persons having only early bronchial reactions. Apart from the effect of IL-5 on the bone marrow, it has also been observed that IL-5 enhances eosinophil maturation in airways of allergic patients [33].

IL-5 can also promote eosinophilic infiltration in bronchial airways due to synergetic effect of IL-5 with other chemoattractants of eosinophils such as eotaxins. The IL-5 role in eosinophil recruitment within the bronchial airways is due to its antiapoptotic action on eosinophils [34]. IL-5 exerts its effect by attachment with IL-5 receptor expressed on eosinophils and basophils. IL-5 receptor is composed of an IL-5-specific α subunit (IL-5Rα) and a nonspecific βc chain that react with IL-5, IL-3, and GM-CSF [35]. The level of IL-5Rα is expressed three times higher on eosinophils than basophils [36].

2.7 Role of IL-33 in pathogenesis

IL-33 is the newly discovered member of cytokine of IL-1 group. Schmitz et al. described IL-33 as a promoter of various type 2-related responses, including cytokine (IL-4, IL-5, and IL-13) and IgE production. In addition to type 2-related response, ST2, the IL-33 receptor, is present on several types of cells engaged in type 2 effector function, including Th2 cells, mast cells, basophils, eosinophils, and ILC2s [37]. Studies in asthma described the supporting role of IL-33 on monocyte development and eosinophil differentiation from the bone marrow [38].

2.8 Role of mast cell pathogenesis

Mast cells are the source of the Th2 cytokines including IL-4 and IL-5 that regulate antibodies' class switching to IgE and eosinophil production, respectively. Mast cells have been observed in higher frequency in asthmatic airways and stimulated by allergen exposure. On activation, mast cells degranulate and secrete their mediators such as histamine and leukotrienes, causing bronchospasm and acute bronchoconstriction by allergen. On the other hand, leukotriene is an essential mediator in airway inflammation and remodeling specifically in symptoms induced by exercise in intrinsic asthma. The granule proteases including tryptase are also released by mast cells. Tryptase is involved in airway remodeling and releases pro-inflammatory chemokine from intracellular matrix [39].

2.9 Role of ILCs in pathogenesis

Innate lymphoid cells (ILCs) are newly discovered immune cells that have lymphoid morphology but deficient in antigen receptor. Type 2 innate lymphoid cells (ILC2) are non-B/non-T cells that release IL-5 and IL-13 on activation by IL-25 and IL-33 and expressed MHC class II high and CD11cdull on their surface. Several studies reported that ILC2 originates from common lymphoid progenitor cells and not from either myeloid or erythroid progenitors, confirming that these cells are of lymphoid origin. ILCs have three different types, ILC1s, ILC2s, and ILC3s, on the basis of identical cytokine profile associated with the helper T subsets Th1, Th2, and Th17, respectively [40]. ILC2s are known to produce type 2 cytokines including IL-4, IL-5, and IL-13 on exposure to allergen, IL-25 and IL-33, and are therefore probable new member in Th2 cell-independent innate type 2 responses. ILC2s can be stimulated by several cytokines especially epithelial cell-derived cytokines IL-25, IL-33, prostaglandin, and leukotriene which have been observed to start ILC2 reaction in both animals and humans [41].

3. Diagnosis

Eosinophilic asthma diagnosis is considered essential in primary, secondary, and tertiary treatments. Typically, general practitioner uses this diagnosis to determine the initialization of inhaled corticosteroids (ICSs). A patient with signs of eosinophilic inflammation is likely to respond to ICSs; however, patients should not be treated with ICSs in the absence of airway eosinophilia. In addition, it is essential to recognize if a patient has airway eosinophilia because those with chronic eosinophilia are susceptible to severe problems and airway remodeling in spite of inhaled or oral corticosteroid treatment. Therefore it must be completely examined [42]. Significantly, all available resources and information are used in all settings to better presume if a person has eosinophilic asthma.

Eosinophilic asthma analysis depends on the confirmation of eosinophilic inflammation in airways of asthmatics, though there is no common diagnostic method. Many procedures can be utilized to diagnose airway eosinophilia in the airways that include induced sputum, bronchial biopsies, blood, and exhaled breath. Generally, airway biopsies or bronchoalveolar lavage (BAL) is principally observed for the analysis of airway inflammation. But for daily clinical use, this method is very invasive. Hence, to determine airway inflammation aseptically in an appropriate and cheap manner. The best recognized and the most common method for testing eosinophilic asthma is the identification of eosinophils in induced sputum [43].

3.1 Bronchial mucosal and BAL eosinophils

The histocytology of a biopsy sample of bronchial tissue could be a diagnostic test to determine the appearance of eosinophils in the submucosa and epithelial cells of air passage. But in daily clinical use, it is impossible to take patients' biopsy due to an invasive method. The interaction between eosinophils is poor in different airway areas because BAL represents eosinophils in the peripheral air passage, while sputum wash and bronchial wash produce a variety of small and adjacent large air passages. Additionally, the analysis of bronchial submucosal and BAL eosinophils is not consistent, so it is difficult to relate results of these tests between laboratories. Roughly, if the tissue and BAL express sufficient amount of eosinophil, possibly they are also increased in sputum. This observation may not be true. More importantly, the number of eosinophils in sputum (airway luminal) is more associated with clinical guidelines for asthma control, like the worsening of symptoms than the numbers of eosinophils in tissue section. This association may not be surprising, provided that eosinophils are triggered as they pass through different areas and are further induced in the lumen of air passage than in tissues [44].

3.2 Eosinophil count in sputum

The advance applications of methods to carefully and accurately induce and assess the sputum have allowed the possibilities to investigate the features of inflammatory process in airway in asthmatics. This brings attention to the heterogeneity of airway inflammation in asthma [45]. Currently, sputum analysis is essentially an extensive and aseptic method for testing the airway inflammation. The analysis of sputum with hypertonic solution of saline is reliable in asthmatics who have just 0.9 L forced expiratory volume in the first second (FEV1) and is effective in almost 80% of asthma patients [46]. The test for the collection, preparation, and determination of cell counts of sputum is easily characterized and organized, and its stability, responsiveness, and validity were explained. The normal values for sputum cell counts were determined, and on the basis of sputum examination, guidelines are available to improve the treatment. However, the eosinophil count in non-asthmatics is 1.2%, while 3% or more sputum eosinophil is usually believed as clinically important. Further investigation is required apart from the complete cell differentiation, probably the levels of biomarkers, like eosinophil-free granules, or the level of protein released from granules (e.g., eosinophil peroxidase) is precise and more significant [47].

3.3 Peripheral blood eosinophil

Eosinophilic counts in a peripheral blood are easily collected and mostly convenient, and still it is deficient in both accuracy and susceptibility. However, some asthmatics perhaps reveal that blood eosinophils rise in those patients who have peripheral eosinophilia. So a proposed association is found with acute asthma signs and decreased pulmonary activity as examined by FEV1 [48]. But in asthma, blood eosinophil counts were not recognized to safely associate with increased eosinophils in sputum. It was shown that eosinophils' quantity (>300/μL) in blood had just 50% positive predictive value in finding the phenotype of an asthma that is on the basis of eosinophil in sputum (>2%). Altogether, these studies show that peripheral blood eosinophilia perhaps is a sign of severe condition in asthma but not constantly associated with sputum eosinophilia.

3.4 Pulmonary function test (PFT)

PFT evaluates volume and rate of airflow that breathe in and out. The FEV1 of exhalation is assessed and compared to the total air volume during forced expiration (forced vital capacity [FVC]). It is an early test for diagnosis of asthma to evaluate airway blockage, disease severity, and reversibility of symptoms. Reduced FEV1, blockage in airflow (lower level of FEV1/FVC), and concavity in FEV loop are expected in patients of asthma [49]. Other PFTs include bronchodilator responsiveness (BDR) test which is predictive of adult-onset asthma. Specific airway resistance (sRaw) analyses by body plethysmography may also be an indicator of early airflow blockage. Hastie et al. reported multiple parameters such as FeNO level, reduced FEV_1, persistent airflow obstruction, total IgE, and blood eosinophil counts in diagnosing eosinophilic asthma [50].

3.5 Exhaled breath condensate (EBC)

EBC is a new, noninvasive test of identifying biological markers, predominantly secreting from the lower part of the airway. EBC is obtained at the time of quiet respiration, as a result of cooling and liquefaction of the air droplets that breathe out [51]. It is a distinct method in detecting molecular pathways related to the respiratory tract. Antus et al. reported lower EBC pH in asthmatic compared with control subjects [52]. Hydrogen peroxide (H_2O_2), an indicator of oxidative stress, was elevated in EBC of patients with asthma. Furthermore, EBC-H_2O_2 concentration is associated with asthma severity and prognosis [53]. Other biomarkers such as CysLTs (LTD_4, LTE_4, and LTC_4), eicosanoids (8-isoprostane and prostaglandin E_2), interleukins (IL-4), and high-sensitivity C-reactive protein (hs-CRP) are found in increased levels in asthma with exercise-induced bronchoconstriction. Serum hs-CRP and fractional exhaled nitric oxide (FeNO) concentration were significantly associated with EBC-hs-CRP levels in patients of asthma [54, 55].

3.6 Fraction of exhaled nitric oxide (FeNO)

Nitric oxide synthase helps in the synthesis of nitric oxide, a reactive molecule that is shown on cells in airway epithelium. In asthma, FeNO analysis by breath assays is usually treated as an aseptic sign of airway inflammation. FeNO analysis is simple, rapid, and noninvasive in contrast to the bronchoscopy and sputum induction. Significantly, it was shown that FeNO quantification perhaps is helpful as a clinical instrument for administering the asthma and managing the disease, but different findings result in some controversy about FeNO efficacy [56]. In a study, more than 90 asthma patients were examined by Smith et al., and they identified that FeNO acts as an effective tool for the withdrawal of inhaled corticosteroid treatment. Tseliou et al. also studied that >19 parts per billion FeNO levels were due to sputum eosinophilia with 78% sensitivity and 73% reactivity in individuals who had mild to acute asthma, while few of them relied on prednisone. Differently, Nair et al. in a clinical trial performed with mepolizumab described that FeNO levels and sputum eosinophil percentages are not associated with asthmatics who relied on prednisone [57].

3.7 Total IgE

IgE plays an important part in allergic asthma. IgE antibodies produced by allergic patients are specific for antigens like pollens and house dust mite, attached with IgE-specific receptors on basophils and mast cells. The connection of IgE molecules stimulates the release of intermediates (arachidonic acid metabolites and histamine) and cytokines (IL-4, tumor necrosis factor alpha, and IL-5) that are important for early- and late-stage allergic response and the associated penetration of eosinophils in the airway. Different findings which have determined a relation between levels of IgE in serum, airway eosinophilic asthma, and anti-IgE treatment were explained, closely related with a remarkable decrease in tissue eosinophils. But in spite of these findings, it is not suggested to use IgE as a biomarker for eosinophilic inflammation. Latest meta-analysis by Korevaar and his fellows, they have described low validity and inadequacy for this biomarker in comparison with FeNO to find sputum eosinophilia [58]. The results were not valid, when comparing blood eosinophils with IgE. Hence, to find eosinophilic asthma, IgE appears to be less effective of all currently available biomarkers.

3.8 Periostin

Periostin is an interleukin-13-regulated matrix protein which is present outside the cells. It was described that periostin promotes the recruitment of allergen-induced eosinophils to the lungs, leading to eosinophil binding to fibronectin. Additionally, it was shown that periostin affects the durability of lung cancer cells due to Akt/PKB pathway; though it has not been examined, maybe it could improve the survival of eosinophils [59].

Generally, periostin is available as an essential biomarker for the detection of eosinophil levels in air passage in asthma patients because of its function in the recruitment of eosinophils in tissue. Jia et al. conducted a study on different parameters that include age, BMI, gender, blood eosinophils, and levels of IgE, FeNO, and periostin in the serum of 59 acute asthmatic cases and demonstrated that airway eosinophilia was best determined by periostin in the serum. The level of periostin (>25 ng/mL) in serum had 93% positive predictive value and 37% negative predictive value for >3% eosinophils in sputum or tissue eosinophilia. In asthma the exact function of periostin is not observed. In addition to function in eosinophilia, animal models propose that perhaps periostin is associated with airway remodeling through growth factor-β switching and can also have supportive part in airway hyperresponsiveness induced by allergen [60].

4. Treatment

The present eosinophilic asthma treatment is introduced with common guideline-based therapy that consists of ICS and bronchodilators that have been thoroughly studied elsewhere [61]. Usually the eosinophil appearance has been linked with susceptibility to corticosteroids, while some eosinophilic asthma patients were identified with subsequent steroid refractory.

Eosinophilic asthma treatment consists of elevated dose of ICS and oral corticosteroids. ICS are primarily used to decrease airway inflammation and mucus hypersecretion, beginning with the reduced strong dosage and increasing to high-dose ICS due to increased intensity. Several severe asthmatics become addicted to corticosteroids. Depending upon toxic corticosteroids for long-term maintenance, treatment perhaps impairs the individuals and may result in corticosteroid resistance [62].

Perhaps many methods which are considered for corticosteroid-resistant asthma have been described in addition to the activation of p38 mitogen-activated protein kinase and inflammatory genes controlled by transcription factor-kB. A p38 mitogen-activated protein kinase is significant to trigger GATA3 (the master

Th2 cytokine transcription factor). Moreover, phosphoinositide 3-kinase (PI3K) controls inflammatory pathways and activates the PI3Kδ isozyme through oxidative stress that can reduce the corticosteroid susceptibility by decreased histone deacetylase 2 (an enzyme marked by theophylline). Further steroid refractory asthma can comprise elevated expression of the alternatively linked variant of the glucocorticoid receptor and elevated formation of macrophage migratory inhibitory factor that can arrest the anti-inflammatory outcomes of corticosteroids [63].

Other factors are under examination for the management of asthma comprised of antagonists focusing on thymic stromal lymphopoietin, IL-25, IL-33, GM-CSF, and chemokine receptor 3 that are expressed on eosinophils [61].

4.1 Biologic therapies

The treatment of refractory eosinophilic asthma includes the drugs that specifically target T helper 2 cytokines as well as anti-IgE, anti-IL-5, and anti-IL-13 monoclonal antibodies [64].

4.1.1 Omalizumab

An IgG1 recombinant humanized monoclonal antibody against IgE is omalizumab. Omalizumab binds with IgE Fc portion, recognizing FcεR1, IgE high-affinity receptors on the top of basophils, and mast cells that result in the downregulation of receptor and suppress the release of inflammatory intermediates. An important function of IgE is to act in allergic response pathophysiology, while omalizumab impairs both early- and late-phase inhaled allergen responses in asthmatics [65]. The previous studies showed a remarkable decrease in eosinophils in airway tissue and induced sputum (8 at baseline in contrast to 1.5 posttreatment) in asthmatics that were treated with omalizumab. Later, it was reported that treatment for 16 weeks reduced the number of eosinophils in blood from 6.2 to 1.3% at baseline [66]. Thus total serum IgE is not applicable for eosinophilic asthma as a diagnostic marker. So, the levels of total IgE in serum should be applied for examining anti-IgE therapy.

The therapy against IgE is effective to eosinophilic asthma treatment in spite of IgE levels. One reason for the observed paradox is that the no response of IgE levels may be associated with the downregulation of FcεR1 by anti-IgE on the surface of basophils, dendritic cells, and mast cells. A decrease in cells that express FcεR1 reduces the intermediate responses of allergen-induced IgE, suppressing the discharge of cytokine and the induction of eosinophil into the airway [67]. Moreover, anti-IgE treatment may assist to reduce the numbers of airway dendritic cells that result in the reduction of Th2 cell differentiation and Th2 cytokines that are required for the recruitment and survival of eosinophils. Thus total IgE in serum may not be related to clinical response or eosinophilic asthma, while omalizumab is useful in the treatment of asthma and decreases the airway eosinophils.

It was studied by Noga et al. that omalizumab is also important as it may have proapoptotic effects on eosinophils [68]. The reduced number of mast cell mediators helps in the stability of eosinophil that may lead to eosinophil apoptosis in individuals that were tested with omalizumab. Particularly, omalizumab is also found as a corticosteroid-sparing drug in persistent eosinophilic pneumonia, a condition that is identified by symmetric lung penetration and the remarkable eosinophil recruitment in blood and BAL fluid [69]. Hence, the outcomes of anti-IgE therapy on lung eosinophilia give more understandings about allergic inflammation mechanisms, which can assist in improving the phenotype-specific analysis.

4.1.2 Targeting IL-5 and interleukin-5 receptor α

The key function of IL-5 in tissues is to stimulate the growth, recruitment, activation, and differentiation of eosinophils. Initial studies described the elevated IL-5 expression in BAL fluid and bronchial biopsies in asthmatic patients. Moreover it was shown that following the allergen confront, IL-5 mRNA was regulated in bronchial mucosa, and the levels were associated with the disease activity. After anti-IL-5 treatment, airway hyperresponsiveness and airway eosinophil assembly after allergen challenge were reduced in animal models [70]. So, there is enough explanation for selecting IL-5 in asthmatics to particularly decrease the eosinophil migration, maturation, and stability that can cause many features of asthma pathogenesis.

4.1.2.1 Mepolizumab

An IgG1-humanized noncomplement-fixing monoclonal antibody is mepolizumab that is specific for human IL-5. Mepolizumab prevents the binding of human IL-5 to the alpha chain of IL-5 receptor complex that is expressed with high affinity on the surface of eosinophil cell. It was shown that in the bronchial mucosa of atopic individuals, anti-IL-5 therapy causes maturational blockage of eosinophil progenitors in the bone marrow and reduces the eosinophil precursors (CD34+ IL-5Rα+) [71]. It is interesting that mepolizumab has different effects in different tissues which results in the complete reduction of eosinophils in sputum and blood exclusively 55% decrease in the bronchial mucosa. It was proposed by Flood-Page et al. that different levels of tissue infiltration could be due to the improved expression or downregulation of IL-5 receptor. Once assembled into the tissue, probably the survival of airway eosinophils depends on IL-3, GM-CSF, or eotaxins.

Two latest findings demonstrate that there could be useful outcome of mepolizumab in certain groups of eosinophilic asthma patients. It was found that double-blind placebo-controlled research consists of 61 cases with a history of chronic acute exacerbations and refractory eosinophilic asthma; following 1-year monthly injections of mepolizumab, a remarkable decrease in exacerbations and recovery in symptom scores were observed in patients treated with mepolizumab [72].

4.1.2.2 Reslizumab

Reslizumab is an anti-IL-5 humanized monoclonal antibody (IgG4), also provided to the eosinophilic asthma patients that were poorly managed [73]. A latest study described a remarkable decrease of eosinophils in sputum, and the respiratory activity improved while relating with inactive drug following monthly 15 weeks of reslizumab therapy (3 mg/kg). The useful results of reslizumab were mostly marked in nasal polyp patients and in those patients who had a maximum level of eosinophils in sputum and blood. Significantly besides the level of eosinophils, the appearance of nasal polyposis can recognize asthma patients that were treated with anti-IL-5.

4.1.2.3 Benralizumab

Benralizumab is an anti-IL-5Rα afucosylated humanized monoclonal antibody, identified on eosinophils and nowadays in Phase II clinical trials. In a prospective Phase II study, the result of one shot of benralizumab (1 mg/kg) that was given intravenously related to the monthly three shots (100 or 200 mg) given subcutaneously or placebo in adult patients of eosinophilic asthma was studied [74]. It was described that following final dose of benralizumab through intravenous and subcutaneous passage helped in the reduction of eosinophil levels in sputum and airway mucosa as well as complete eosinophil count arrest in peripheral blood and bone marrow for up to 28 days.

4.1.3 Targeting interleukin-4 and interleukin-4 receptor α

IL-4 and IL-13 are essential cytokines in the pathogenesis of atopic disease and allergic asthma. These are expressed by basophils, innate lymphoid cells, mast cells, and Th2 cells. IL-4 is important for various asthma characteristics that include mucus formation, switching of B-cell isotypes, and differentiation of Th2 cells. IL-4 and IL-13 transmit signal inside the cells by two different overlapped heterodimeric receptors which are part of IL-Rα [75]. Receptor attachment is triggered by a typical signaling pathway, signal transducer and activator of transcription 6 (STAT-6), that is important for the production of Th2 inflammation, an asthma feature. Significantly, eotaxins help in eosinophilic induction as well as rely on IL-4 or IL-13 for the stimulation of STAT-6. At present many drugs are under examination that use IL-4/IL-13/STAT-6 pathway.

4.1.3.1 Pascolizumab

Pascolizumab is a human-based IL-4 monoclonal antibody that was considered in animal studies as well as Phase I and II clinical trials. Pascolizumab was strongly accepted in Phase I clinical trial with mild to moderate asthma in adult patients; anyhow following Phase II trial on a large scale was stopped because it was unsuccessful to express the clinical results in symptomatic individuals who were steroid immature [76].

4.1.3.2 Altrakincept

Altrakincept is an artificial humanized antagonist IL-4Rα that inhibits the penetration of airway eosinophils and hypersecretion of mucus in a mouse model when managed during allergen challenges. One dose of the medicine improves the pulmonary activity and disease problems in Phase I and II trials [77].

4.1.3.3 Pitrakinra

Pitrakinra is an antagonist, which targets the heterodimeric receptor of IL-4 and IL-13 cytokines, comprises the subunits IL-4Rα and IL-13Rα1. Pitrakinra suppressed the early-stage and late-stage reactions produced by allergen when managed by the subcutaneous or inhaled passage [78].

4.1.3.4 Dupilumab

A humanized monoclonal antibody to the IL-4Rα subunit is dupilumab, currently described in a follow-up study analysis [79]. It was studied that 104 subjects with mild to acute persistent asthma and eosinophilia were separated to gain subcutaneously a single dose (300 mg) of dupilumab or placebo in a week for 12 weeks. In the treated group, this study developed a remarkable recovery in lung function related to the decrease in asthma inflammation as long-acting beta-agonists, and received steroids were absorbed. In addition, the significant modifications from basic standards in Th2-related indicators, as well as FeNO,

IgE, chemokine ligand 17, and chemokine ligand 26 (eotaxin-3), were found in the group of dupilumab by 12 weeks. The levels of blood and sputum eosinophils were not dissimilar following dupilumab therapy, while there were less number of people who give sputum, so statistical examination was excluded. Generally, identifying the IL-4Rα signaling (that also stimulates IL-13 signaling) acts as a good therapeutic approach for eosinophilic asthma.

4.1.4 Targeting IL-13

An important part of IL-13 in airway eosinophilic induction in a way depends on the combined function of IL-5 and eotaxin in mouse models. Additionally, many studies demonstrate that IL-13 is important for corticosteroid protection in asthma. In a study on animals, IL-13 inhibition procedures have described reduction in airway hyperresponsiveness, inflammation caused by environmental immunogen, and remodeling of airways [80]. Thus nowadays, pharmaceuticals that target this cytokine are under examination in those who have refractory eosinophilic asthma due to steroids.

4.1.4.1 Anrukinzumab

Anrukinzumab is a complete human IL-13-targeted antibody. In Phase II clinical trial, its effects have shown a decrease in late asthmatic responses produced by allergen after two doses (2 mg/kg) that were given subcutaneously for 2 weeks [80].

4.1.4.2 Lebrikizumab

Lebrikizumab is a humanized anti-IL-13 monoclonal antibody. In a latest study, lebrikizumab was investigated in 219 adults with weakly controlled asthma against long-acting beta-agonists and ICSs [81]. Consequently, the treated group after 12 weeks of therapy has improved FEV1, while high pretreatment with serum periostin levels has more good effects in patients. In post hoc examination, it was interesting that high FeNO and Th2 markers which include CCL13 (human monocyte chemoattractant protein-4), peripheral eosinophilia, CCL17, and total IgE levels were further related with a significant decrease in the levels of acute problems in lebrikizumab-treated cases relative to placebo.

4.1.4.3 Tralokinumab

Tralokinumab is another antibody against IL-13, also effective in Phase II study in improving the lung activity of individuals with moderate to acute asthma [81].

5. Conclusions

In conclusion, asthma is a heterogeneous condition with several phenotypes and endotypes on the basis of different immunopathogenic mechanisms such as underlying inflammation, environmental factors, and disease severity. Understanding of distinct phenotypes with specific pathophysiology is essential for management of patients with eosinophilic asthma. Categorization of asthma into eosinophilic and non-eosinophilic subphenotypes depends on the difference in cells involved in inflammation of respiratory airway. Generally, eosinophilic inflammation has been linked with extrinsic (allergic) asthma with Th2-type response, but now eosinophils have also been observed in the airways of nonallergic (intrinsic) asthma. The development of new biological therapies like monoclonal immunoglobulin and small particles that block IgE, interleukins of Th2 type, and particular inflammatory factors has improved the knowledge about the immunopathogenesis of this phenotype and emphasizes the significance of individual-directed treatment. For doctors, it is essential to early recognize eosinophilic patients because this phenotype may need patient-directed therapies to prevent worsening of asthma symptoms.

Acknowledgements

I am thankful to the University Institute of Medical Laboratory department, the University of Lahore, for being helpful. My deepest gratitude to Prof. Dr. Syed Amir Gillani (Dean of FAHS) and Prof. Dr. Nazar Ullah Raja (Head of the Department of University Institute of Medical Laboratory Technology) for their support.

Conflict of interest

No financial support and no other potential conflict of interest relevant to this chapter were reported.

Acronyms and abbreviations

FcεR1	Fc epsilon receptor 1
GINA	Global Initiative for Asthma
WHO	World Health Organization
IL	interleukin
Th2 cells	type 2 helper T cells
ILCs2 cells	type 2 innate lymphoid cells
LPS	lipopolysaccharides
PGD2	prostaglandin D2
TGF	transforming growth factor

Author details

Bushra Mubarak[1*], Huma Shakoor[1] and Fozia Masood[2]

1 University Institute of Medical Laboratory Technology, The University of Lahore, Lahore, Pakistan

2 Faculty of Pharmacy, The University of Lahore, Lahore, Pakistan

*Address all correspondence to: bushra.mubarik@yahoo.com

References

[1] Anandan C, Nurmatov U, van Schyack OCP, Sheikh A. Is the prevalence of asthma declining? Systematic review of epidemiological studies. Allergy. 2010;**65**:152-167

[2] Mubarak B, Afzal N, Javaid K, Talib R, Aslam R, Latif W. Frequency of HLA DQβ1*0201 and DQβ1*0301 alleles and total serum IgE in patients with bronchial asthma: A pilot study from Pakistan. Iranian Journal of Allergy, Asthma, and Immunology. 2017;**16**(4):313-320

[3] Kalliomaki M, Kirjavainen P, Eerola E, et al. Distinct patterns of neonatal gut flora in infants in whom atopy was and was not developing. The Journal of Allergy and Clinical Immunology. 2001;**107**:129-134

[4] Devouassoux G, Saxon A, Metcalfe DD, et al. Chemical constituents of diesel exhaust particles induce IL-4 production and histamine release by human basophil. The Journal of Allergy and Clinical Immunology. 2002;**109**:847-853

[5] Riedler J, Braun-Fahlander C, Eden W, et al. Exposure to farming in early life and development of asthma and allergy: A cross sectional survey. Lancet. 2001;**358**:1129-1133

[6] Agache I, Akdis C, Jutel M, et al. Untangling asthma phenotypes and endotypes. Allergy. 2012;**67**:835-846

[7] Peters SP. Asthma phenotypes: Nonallergic (intrinsic) asthma. The Journal of Allergy and Clinical Immunology. 2014;**2**(6):650-652

[8] Bateman ED, Hurd SS, Barnes PJ, Bousquet J, FitzGerald M, Gibson P, et al. Global strategy for asthma management and prevention: GINA executive summary. The European Respiratory Journal. 2008;**31**:143-178

[9] American Thoracic Society. Proceedings of the ATS workshop on refractory asthma. Current understanding, recommendations, and unanswered questions. American Journal of Respiratory and Critical Care Medicine. 2000;**162**:2341-2351. Available from: https://www.ncbi.nlm.nih.gov/pubmed/11112161

[10] Bousquet J, Mantzouranis E, Cruz AA, et al. Uniform definition of asthma severity, control, and exacerbations: Document presented for the World Health Organization Consultation on Severe Asthma. The Journal of Allergy and Clinical Immunology. 2010;**126**:926-938

[11] Szczeklik A, Stevenson DD. Aspirin-induced asthma: Advances in pathogenesis, diagnosis, and management. The Journal of Allergy and Clinical Immunology. 2003;**111**:913-921

[12] Haldar P, Pavord I, Shaw D, Berry M, Thomas M, Brightling C, et al. Cluster analysis and clinical asthma phenotypes. American Journal of Respiratory and Critical Care Medicine. 2008;**1**:218-224

[13] De Groot JC, Brinke AT, Bel EHD. Management of the patient with eosinophilic asthma: A new era begins. ERJ Open Research. 2015;**1**(1):00024

[14] Xie M, Wenzel SE. A global perspective in asthma: From phenotype to endotype. Chinese Medical Journal. 2013;**126**(1):166-174

[15] Raundhal M, Morse C, Khare A, et al. High IFN-gamma and low SLPI mark severe asthma in mice and humans. The Journal of Clinical Investigation. 2015;**125**(8):3037-3050

[16] Steinke JW, Borish L. Factors driving the aspirin exacerbated respiratory disease phenotype.

American Journal of Rhinology & Allergy. 2015;**29**(1):35-40

[17] Miranda C, Busacker A, Balzar S, Trudeau J, Wenzel SE. Distinguishing severe asthma phenotypes: Role of age at onset and eosinophilic inflammation. The Journal of Allergy and Clinical Immunology. 2004;**113**:101-108

[18] Yu S, Kim HY, Chang YJ, Dekruyff RH, Umetsu DT. Innate lymphoid cells and asthma. Journal of Allergy and Clinical Immunology. 2014;**133**(4):943-950

[19] Su Z, Lin J, Lu F, et al. Potential autocrine regulation of interleukin-33/ST2 signaling of dendritic cells in allergic inflammation. Mucosal Immunology. 2013;**6**(5):921-930

[20] Pawankar R, Hayashi M, Yamanishi S, Igarashi T. The paradigm of cytokine networks in allergic airway inflammation. Current Opinion in Allergy and Clinical Immunology. 2015;**15**(1):41-48

[21] Hallstrand TS, Henderson WR. An update on the role of leukotrienes in asthma. Current Opinion in Allergy and Clinical Immunology. 2010;**10**(1):60-66

[22] Hall S, Agrawal DK. Key mediators in the immunopathogenesis of allergic asthma. International Immunopharmacology. 2014;**23**(1):316-329

[23] Lambrecht BN, Hammad H. The immunology of asthma. Nature Immunology. 2014;**16**(1):45-56

[24] Brusselle GG, Maes T, Bracke KR. Eosinophilic airway inflammation in nonallergic asthma. Nature Medicine. 2013;**19**(8):977-979

[25] Walsh GM. Targeting eosinophils in asthma: Current and future state of cytokine- and chemokine-directed monoclonal therapy. Expert Review of Clinical Immunology. 2010;**6**:701-704

[26] Schwartz N, Grossman A, Levy Y, Schwarz Y. Correlation between eosinophil count and methacholine challenge test in asymptomatic subjects. The Journal of Asthma. 2012;**49**:336-341

[27] Fattouh R, Jordana M. TGF-beta, eosinophils and IL-13 in allergic airway remodeling: A critical appraisal with therapeutic considerations. Inflammation & Allergy Drug Targets. 2008;**7**:224-236

[28] Molet S, Hamid Q, Davoine F, et al. IL-17 is increased in asthmatic airways and induces human bronchial fibroblasts to produce cytokines. The Journal of Allergy and Clinical Immunology. 2001;**108**:430-438

[29] Feltis BN, Wignarajah D, Zheng L, et al. Increased vascular endothelial growth factor and receptors: Relationship to angiogenesis in asthma. American Journal of Respiratory and Critical Care Medicine. 2006;**173**:1201-1207

[30] Sonar SS, Ehmke M, Marsh LM, Dietze J, Dudda JC, Conrad ML, et al. Clara cells drive eosinophil accumulation in allergic asthma. The European Respiratory Journal. 2012;**39**:429-438

[31] Schuijs MJ, Willart MA, Hammad H, et al. Cytokine targets in airway inflammation. Current Opinion in Pharmacology. 2013;**13**:351-361

[32] Jacobsen EA, Zellner KR, Colbert D, Lee NA, Lee JJ. Eosinophils regulate dendritic cells and Th2 pulmonary immune responses following allergen provocation. Journal of Immunology. 2011;**187**:6059-6068

[33] Dorman SC, Efthimiadis A, Babirad I, et al. Sputum CD34+ IL-5Rα+ cells increase after allergen: Evidence for in situ eosinophilopoiesis. American Journal of Respiratory and Critical Care Medicine. 2004;**169**(5):573-577

[34] Ilmarinen P, Moilanen E, Kankaanranta H. Regulation of spontaneous eosinophil apoptosis—A neglected area of importance. Journal of Cell Death. 2014;7:1-9

[35] Brusselle GG, Maes T, Bracke KR. Eosinophilic airway inflammation in non-allergic asthma. Nature Medicine. 2013;**19**(8):977-979

[36] Kolbeck R, Kozhich A, Koike M, Peng L, Andersson C, Damschroder M, et al. MEDI-563, a humanized anti-IL-5 receptor alpha mAb with enhanced antibody-dependent cell-mediated cytotoxicity function. The Journal of Allergy and Clinical Immunology. 2010;**125**:1344-1353

[37] Neill DR, Wong SH, Bellosi A, Flynn RJ, Daly M, Langford TK, et al. Nuocytes represent a new innate effector leukocyte that mediates type-2 immunity. Nature. 2010;**464**:1367-1370

[38] Dyer KD, Percopo CM, Rosenberg HF. IL-33 promotes eosinophilia in vivo and antagonizes IL-5-dependent eosinophil hematopoiesis ex vivo. Immunology Letters. 2013;**150**:41-47

[39] Klein Wolterink RG, Kleinjan A, van Nimwegen M, Bergen I, de Bruijn M, Levani Y, et al. Pulmonary innate lymphoid cells are major producers of IL-5 and IL-13 in murine models of allergic asthma. European Journal of Immunology. 2012;**42**(5):1106-1116

[40] Barlow JL, McKenzie AN. Type-2 innate lymphoid cells in human allergic disease. Current Opinion in Allergy and Clinical Immunology. 2014;**14**(5):397-403

[41] Chang JE, Doherty TA, Baum R, Broide D. Prostaglandin D2 regulates human type 2 innate lymphoid cell chemotaxis. The Journal of Allergy and Clinical Immunology. 2014;**133**(3):899-901

[42] Jayaram L, Pizzichini MM, Cook RJ, et al. Determining asthma treatment by monitoring sputum cell counts: Effect on exacerbations. The European Respiratory Journal. 2006;**27**(3):483-494

[43] In 'T Veen JCCM, De Gouw HWFM, Smits HH, et al. Repeatability of cellular and soluble markers of inflammation in induced sputum from patients with asthma. The European Respiratory Journal. 1996;**9**(12):2441-2447

[44] Persson C, Uller L. Primary lysis of eosinophils as a major mode of activation of eosinophils in human diseased tissues. Nature Reviews. Immunology. 2013;**13**(12):902

[45] D'Silva L, Hassan N, Wang HY, et al. Heterogeneity of bronchitis in airway diseases in tertiary care clinical practice. Canadian Respiratory Journal. 2011;**18**(3):144-148

[46] Persson C, Uller L. Theirs but to die and do: Primary lysis of eosinophils and free eosinophil granules in asthma. American Journal of Respiratory and Critical Care Medicine. 2014;**189**(6):628-633

[47] Ulrik CS. Peripheral eosinophil counts as a marker of disease activity in intrinsic and extrinsic asthma. Clinical and Experimental Allergy. 1995;**25**:820-827

[48] Silkoff PE, Lent AM, Busacker AA, et al. Exhaled nitric oxide identifies the persistent eosinophilic phenotype in severe refractory asthma. The Journal of Allergy and Clinical Immunology. 2005;**116**:1249-1255

[49] Pellegrino R, Viegi G, Brusasco V, et al. Interpretative strategies for lung function tests. The European Respiratory Journal. 2005;**26**:948-968

[50] Hastie AT, Moore WC, Li H, et al. Biomarker surrogates do not

accurately predict sputum eosinophil and neutrophil percentages in asthmatic subjects. The Journal of Allergy and Clinical Immunology. 2013;**132**:72-80

[51] Horvath I, Hunt J, Barnes PJ, et al. Exhaled breath condensate: Methodological recommendations and unresolved questions. The European Respiratory Journal. 2005;**26**(3):523-548

[52] Antus B, Barta I, Kullmann T, et al. Assessment of exhaled breath condensate pH in exacerbations of asthma and chronic obstructive pulmonary disease: A longitudinal study. AJRCCM. 2010;**182**(12):1492-1497

[53] Teng Y, Sun P, Zhang J, et al. Hydrogen peroxide in exhaled breath condensate in patients with asthma: A promising biomarker? Chest. 2011;**140**(1):108-116

[54] Bikov A, Gajdocsi R, Huszar E, et al. Exercise increases exhaled breath condensate cysteinyl leukotriene concentration in asthmatic patients. The Journal of Asthma. 2010;**47**(9):1057-1062

[55] Zietkowski Z, Tomasiak-Lozowska MM, Skiepko R, Mroczko B, Szmitkowski M, Bodzenta-Lukaszyk A. High-sensitivity C-reactive protein in the exhaled breath condensate and serum in stable and unstable asthma. Respiratory Medicine. 2009;**103**(3):379-385

[56] Nair P, Pizzichini MM, Kjarsgaard M, et al. Mepolizumab for prednisone-dependent asthma with sputum eosinophilia. The New England Journal of Medicine. 2009;**360**:985-993

[57] Korevaar DA, Westerhof GA, Wang J, et al. Diagnostic accuracy of minimally invasive markers for detection of airway eosinophilia in asthma: A systematic review and meta-analysis. The Lancet Respiratory Medicine. 2015;**3**(4):290-300

[58] Ouyang G, Liu M, Ruan K, Song G, Mao Y, Bao S. Upregulated expression of periostin by hypoxia in non-small-cell lung cancer cells promotes cell survival via the Akt/PKB pathway. Cancer Letters. 2009;**281**:213-219

[59] Gordon ED, Sidhu SS, Wang ZE, et al. A protective role for periostin and TGF-beta in IgE-mediated allergy and airway hyperresponsiveness. Clinical and Experimental Allergy. 2012;**42**:144-155

[60] Pelaia G, Vatrella A, Maselli R. The potential of biologics for the treatment of asthma. Nature Reviews. Drug Discovery. 2012;**11**:958-972

[61] Barnes PJ. Severe asthma: Advances in current management and future therapy. The Journal of Allergy and Clinical Immunology. 2012;**129**:48-59

[62] Walford HH, Doherty TA. Diagnosis and management of eosinophilic asthma: A US perspective. Journal of Asthma and Allergy. 2014;**7**:53-65

[63] Barnes PJ, Adcock IM. Glucocorticoid resistance in inflammatory diseases. Lancet. 2009;**373**:1905-1917

[64] Noga O, Hanf G, Brachmann I, et al. Effect of omalizumab treatment on peripheral eosinophil and T-lymphocyte function in patients with allergic asthma. The Journal of Allergy and Clinical Immunology. 2006;**117**:1493-1499

[65] Noga O, Hanf G, Kunkel G. Immunological and clinical changes in allergic asthmatics following treatment with omalizumab. International Archives of Allergy and Immunology. 2003;**131**:46-52

[66] Holgate S, Casale T, Wenzel S, Bousquet J, Deniz Y, Reisner C. The anti-inflammatory effects of omalizumab confirm the central role of IgE in allergic inflammation.

The Journal of Allergy and Clinical Immunology. 2005;**115**:459-465

[67] Kaya H, Gumus S, Ucar E, et al. Omalizumab as a steroid-sparing agent in chronic eosinophilic pneumonia. Chest. 2012;**142**:513-516

[68] Garlisi CG, Kung TT, Wang P, et al. Effects of chronic anti-interleukin-5 monoclonal antibody treatment in a murine model of pulmonary inflammation. American Journal of Respiratory Cell and Molecular Biology. 1999;**20**:248-255

[69] Menzies-Gow A, Flood-Page P, Sehmi R, et al. Anti-IL-5 (mepolizumab) therapy induces bone marrow eosinophil maturational arrest and decreases eosinophil progenitors in the bronchial mucosa of atopic asthmatics. The Journal of Allergy and Clinical Immunology. 2003;**111**:714-719

[70] Haldar P, Brightling CE, Hargadon B, et al. Mepolizumab and exacerbations of refractory eosinophilic asthma. The New England Journal of Medicine. 2009;**360**:973-984

[71] Castro M, Mathur S, Hargreave F, et al. Reslizumab for poorly controlled, eosinophilic asthma: A randomized, placebo-controlled study. American Journal of Respiratory and Critical Care Medicine. 2011;**184**:1125-1132

[72] Laviolette M, Gossage DL, Gauvreau G, et al. Effects of benralizumab on airway eosinophils in asthmatic patients with sputum eosinophilia. The Journal of Allergy and Clinical Immunology. 2013;**132**(5):1086-1096

[73] Ingram JL, Kraft M. IL-13 in asthma and allergic disease: Asthma phenotypes and targeted therapies. The Journal of Allergy and Clinical Immunology. 2012;**130**:829-842

[74] Hart TK, Blackburn MN, Brigham-Burke M, et al. Preclinical efficacy and safety of pascolizumab (SB 240683): A humanized anti-interleukin-4 antibody with therapeutic potential in asthma. Clinical and Experimental Immunology. 2002;**130**:93-100

[75] Borish LC, Nelson HS, Corren J, et al. Efficacy of soluble IL-4 receptor for the treatment of adults with asthma. The Journal of Allergy and Clinical Immunology. 2001;**107**:963-970

[76] Wenzel S, Wilbraham D, Fuller R, Getz EB, Longphre M. Effect of an interleukin-4 variant on late phase asthmatic response to allergen challenge in asthmatic patients: Results of two phase 2a studies. Lancet. 2007;**370**:1422-1431

[77] Wenzel S, Ford L, Pearlman D, et al. Dupilumab in persistent asthma with elevated eosinophil levels. The New England Journal of Medicine. 2013;**368**:2455-2466

[78] Yang G, Volk A, Petley T, et al. Anti-IL-13 monoclonal antibody inhibits airway hyperresponsiveness, inflammation and airway remodeling. Cytokine. 2004;**28**:224-232

[79] Gauvreau GM, Boulet LP, Cockcroft DW, et al. Effects of interleukin-13 blockade on allergen-induced airway responses in mild atopic asthma. American Journal of Respiratory and Critical Care Medicine. 2011;**183**:1007-1014

[80] Corren J, Lemanske RF, Hanania NA, et al. Lebrikizumab treatment in adults with asthma. The New England Journal of Medicine. 2011;**365**:1088-1098

[81] Piper E, Brightling C, Niven R, et al. A phase II placebo-controlled study of tralokinumab in moderate-to-severe asthma. The European Respiratory Journal. 2013;**41**:330-338

Chapter 7

Role of Various Mediators in Inflammation of Asthmatic Airways

Poonam Arora and S.H. Ansari

Abstract

The degree of airway inflammation is directly related to asthma severity and associated hyper-responsiveness. Airway inflammation is categorized into three types: (a) acute asthmatic inflammation featured by early recruitment of cells into the airways, (b) subacute asthmatic inflammation involving activation of recruited cells in continual inflammation, and (c) chronic inflammation characterized by cellular damage. T-helper lymphocytes, the key factor in the pathogenesis of bronchial asthma, induce B cells to synthesize and secrete IgE through production of IL-4 and induce eosinophil-mediated inflammation. Mediators such as histamine, PG, leukotrienes, and kinins contract airway smooth muscle, increase microvascular leakage, increase airway mucus secretion, and attract other inflammatory cells into airway epithelia that initiate mucociliary clearance signaling pathways through special Toll-like receptor 4 expressed on epithelial cells activated by allergic and infectious triggers. These cells form barrier against mechanical stress, oxidant stress, allergens, pollutants, infectious agents, and leakage of endogenous solutes. Various adhesion molecules and costimulatory factors also promote infiltration of inflammatory cells at the site of inflammation.

Keywords: airway inflammation, hyper-responsiveness, bronchial asthma, T-helper lymphocytes, mediators

1. Introduction

The inflammatory response in asthmatic airways is a complex interplay between respiratory epithelium and immune system. The drive for a chronic inflammatory response initiates with production of bioactive mediators from airway epithelium, which attracts, activates, and recruits the inflammatory cells into lung airways. Infiltrated cells augment inflammatory response through the release of other biochemical mediators. The inflammatory mediators released by these cells are the effectors of chronic inflammation including cytokines classified into lymphokines or immunomodulatory cytokines released by T-helper cells, proinflammatory cytokines that promote and amplify the inflammatory response, chemokines that are chemoattractants for leukocytes, growth factors that promote cell survival, and eicosanoid lipid mediators that have multiple effects in the airway. The products released from leukocytes and epithelial cells induce bronchospasm, damage the epithelium, stimulate airway cells, and recruit additional leukocytes creating a cycle of inflammation that becomes chronic. In acute cases of allergen exposure, mast cells can provide an early source of proinflammatory mediators such as IL-4 and IL-5. Episodes of acute inflammatory reactions are often accompanied by an underlying chronic inflammation even in the absence of continuous allergen exposure.

2. Airway inflammation in asthma

The degree of airway inflammation and corresponding airway hyper-responsiveness (AHR) is related to clinical symptoms in asthma. Asthmatic inflammation is categorized into three types: (a) acute asthmatic inflammation featured by early recruitment of cells into the airways, (b) subacute asthmatic inflammation involving activation of recruited cells in continual inflammation, and (c) chronic inflammation characterized by cellular damage. Various types of biogenic mediators that play an important part in inflammatory process in asthmatic airways are given in **Figure 1**.

2.1 Cells

2.1.1 Eosinophils

Eosinophil infiltration is a characteristic feature of asthmatic airway inflammation that plays a central role in asthma. Allergen inhalation results in a marked increase in eosinophil count in bronchoalveolar (BAL) fluid at the time of the late asthma response with a decrease in peripheral eosinophil counts with the appearance of eosinophil precursors in the circulation. Recruitment of eosinophils to airways is mediated by interleukin (IL)-13, histamine, prostaglandin type 2, and chemokines, such as RANTES (regulated on activation T-cell expressed and secreted), eotaxins, and macrophage chemotactic protein (MCP)-4, expressed in epithelial cells [1, 2].

2.1.2 Neutrophils

Neutrophils are predominantly observed in the airways and sputum of patients with severe asthma [3], especially during acute exacerbations of asthma and in some patients with long-lasting or corticosteroids dependent or unresponsive to inhaled steroids. They are recruited through Th17 pathways and lead to increased concentrations of IL-8 in sputum, which in turn may be due to the increased levels

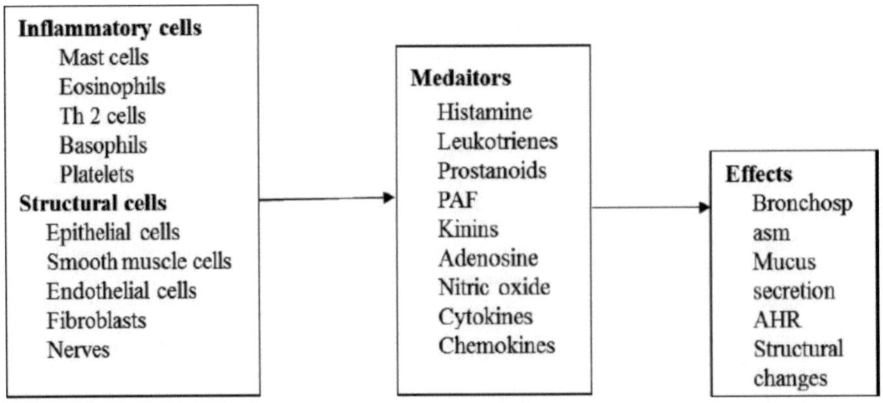

Figure 1.
Inflammatory mediators in asthma.

of oxidative stress in severe asthma [4]. Neutrophils contribute to BHR and airway inflammation through the release of mediators like PAF, thromboxanes, and leukotrienes and tissue damage through secretion of proteases and oxygen radicals [5].

2.1.3 Macrophages

Macrophages, derived from blood monocytes, extend inflammatory process in asthma through production of a variety of cytokines, after being activated by allergen via low-affinity IgE receptors (FceRII) [6]. Macrophages may both increase and decrease inflammation, depending on the stimulus. Alveolar macrophages normally have a suppressive effect on lymphocyte function, but this may get impaired in asthma after allergen exposure [7]. Macrophages secrete an anti-inflammatory protein IL-10 which is reduced in alveolar macrophages from patients with asthma [8]. Macrophages may, therefore, play an important anti-inflammatory role, by preventing the development of allergic inflammation [9].

2.1.4 Mast cells

Mast cells are central to the development of type I hypersensitivity reaction. Mast cells are bone marrow-derived cells widely distributed in the body predominantly near blood vessels, subepithelial cells and nerves, mucosal lining of the gut, and upper and lower respiratory tract. Increased numbers of degranulated mast cells have been found in asthma exacerbation [10]. Mast cells contain membrane-bound granules filled with biologically active mediators.

After re-exposure, mast cells get activated by cross-linking of high-affinity IgE Fc receptors present on mast cell surface or by stimuli such as C5a and C3a (anaphylatoxins) and release a wide variety of mediators that result in acute bronchospasm or perpetuate underlying inflammation through cytokines [11]. Mast cells are an important source of histamine, cysteinyl leukotrienes, prostaglandins, cytokines, and platelet-activating factor, after getting activated by binding of stem cell factor to the surface receptor c-kit, IgE cross-linking, or binding of tyrosine kinase [12], and the process is called degranulation of mast cells (**Figure 2**).

2.1.5 T-lymphocytes

Several types of T-lymphocytes (especially, Th1, Th2, Th9, and Th17) play an important role in coordinating the inflammatory response in asthma through release of a number of cytokines. Traditionally, Th2 cells have been thought to predominate, with characteristic raised levels of IL-4, IL-5, and IL-13. High proportion of T_H1 cells that can develop under the influence of IL-18 and interferon γ (IFN-γ) associated with further production of IFN-γ is found in some asthmatics. Th17 cells, expressing IL-17, also play an unusual role in asthmatic patients [13]. Th17 are CD4-positive T cells and result in neutrophils influx. Th9 levels are raised in people with atopy cells, secrete IL-9, and promote allergic responses, probably through activation of mast cells. T-regulatory cells, characterized by secretion of transforming growth factor β (TGF-β) and IL-10, are thought to be important because of their role in blunting atopic responses [14].

2.1.6 B-lymphocytes

B cells are important in asthma associated with atopy because they produce IgE. Their survival is supported by IL-5 and a B-cell-activating factor. B cells need to bind to T cells under the influence of IL-4 or IL-13. Secreted IgE are primarily bound through the

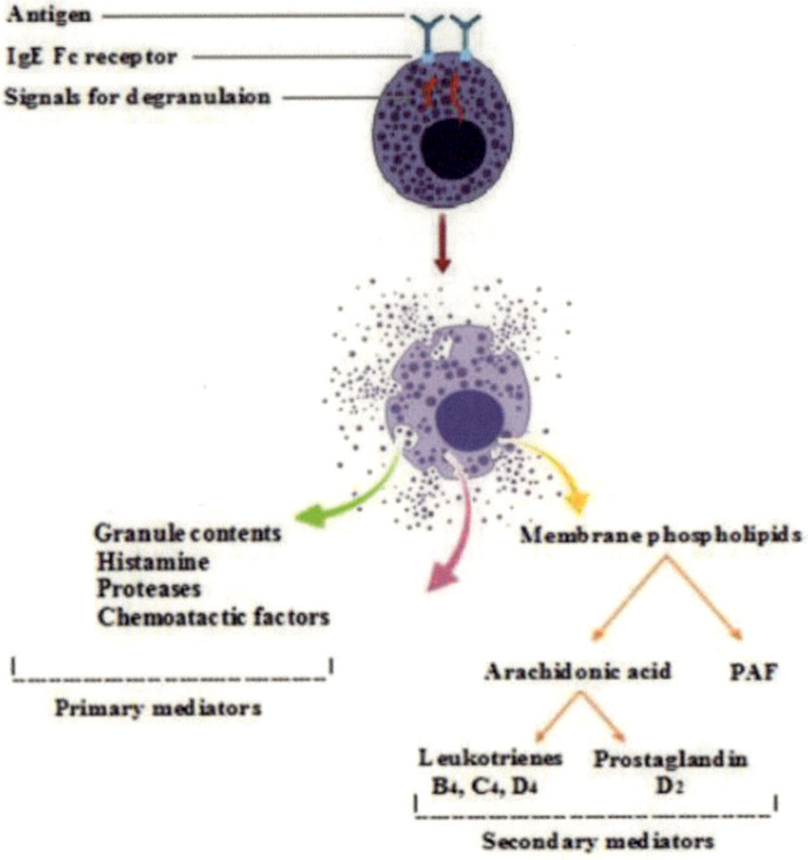

Figure 2.
Activation of mast cells and release of mediators in allergic asthma.

high-affinity Fc receptors on mast cells and basophils, and when cross-linked by aeroallergen, it causes these cells to degranulate and release their mediators [15].

2.1.7 Innate lymphoid cells

ILCs are a family of immune cells that are defined by several features including the absence of recombination-activating gene (RAG)-dependent rearranged antigen receptors, their lymphoid morphology, as well as lack of myeloid phenotypic markers and are therefore called cell lineage marker-negative (Lin−) cells. These ILCs are present in the skin, adipose tissues, mesenteric lymph nodes, tonsils, and spleen and mediate inflammatory pathways in various diseases of the lungs and skin. ILCs are classified into three groups according to their transcription factors and cytokine production profile that resembles T-helper (TH) cell subsets [16]. Among these cells, group 2 innate lymphoid cells (ILC2s) are known to play a role in pathogenesis of type 2 inflammatory diseases of the lungs and skin such as asthma and atopic dermatitis [17]. They have the capacity to produce type 2 (T_H2) cytokines and interact with both immune and nonimmune cell populations in the local tissue environment. ILC1s produce T_H1 inflammatory cytokines, particularly IFN-γ and tumor necrosis factor (TNF-α). They play their role in the pathogenesis of chronic obstructive pulmonary disease (COPD) and human inflammatory bowel (IBD). ILCs generally differentiate into macrophages and granulocytes while stimulating eosinophils and producing Th2 cytokines [18].

2.1.8 Airway epithelial cells

Airway epithelial cells play an important role in mucociliary clearance signaling through special receptors Toll-like receptor 4 expressed on epithelial cells activated by allergic and infectious triggers. These cells form barrier against mechanical stress, oxidant stress, allergens, pollutants, infectious agents, and leakage of endogenous solutes. In asthma, epithelial cell-derived cytokines and chemokines (including IL-25, IL-33, thymic stromal lymphopoietin [TSLP], and granulocyte-macrophage colony-stimulating factor [GM-CSF]) signal effector cells (including basophils, eosinophils, mast cells, and lymphocytes) and dendritic cells are of importance in developing characteristic asthmatic immune response patterns to various types of allergic stimuli [19].

2.1.9 Dendritic cells

Like airway epithelial cells, pulmonary dendritic cells are also directly exposed to the external environment. These dendritic cells act as antigen-presenting cells and are directly stimulated by allergens or infectious agents directly after binding with recognition receptors or indirectly stimulated by airway epithelial cells (by mediators such as IL-25, IL-33, GM-CSF); dendritic cells can recruit eosinophils in allergen-presenting regions [20]. Dendritic cells are also found to effect T-cell differentiation and generate Th2 response commonly seen in atopic asthma [21].

2.2 Adhesion molecules

These molecules promote infiltration of inflammatory cells at the site of inflammation, recruitment of leukocytes from vascular lumen to tissues, and cell activation [22]. Adhesion molecules are upregulated in allergic inflammation and play a critical role in pathogenesis inflammation. More than 35 adhesion molecules have been identified, for example, integrins, immunoglobulin supergene family, selectins, and carbohydrate ligands including ICAM-1 and VCAM-1.

2.3 Costimulatory factors

A number of costimulatory factors are known to play an important role in the development of immunity such as inducible costimulator (ICOS) and ligand for ICOS. ICOS is known to regulate production of Th2 cytokines and to have a significant role in lung mucosal inflammatory responses [23, 24].

2.4 Inflammatory mediators

A number of mediators that account for pathophysiological features of allergic diseases have been implicated in asthma. Mediators such as histamine, PG, leukotrienes, and kinins contract airway smooth muscle, increase microvascular leakage, increase airway mucus secretion, and attract other inflammatory cells.

2.4.1 Histamine

Histamine was the first mediator known to be implicated in pathophysiology of asthma. Histamine is synthesized and released by mast cells and basophils in the airways. Histamine causes mucus secretion and bronchoconstriction which is partially mediated by vagal cholinergic reflex. Histamine also acts as a chemoattractant for eosinophils and activates eosinophils [25].

2.4.2 Leukotrienes

The cysteinyl leukotrienes, LTC_4, LTD_4, and LTE_4, are eicosanoids derived from arachidonic acid by 5-LOX (lipoxygenase) pathway. They are potent constrictors of human airway and have been reported to increase AHR and play an important role in asthma [3]. They constitute the slow-reacting substance of anaphylaxis. [26]. Potent LTD_4 antagonists protect (by 50%) against exercise- and allergen-induced bronchoconstriction, suggesting that leukotrienes contribute to bronchoconstrictor responses.

2.4.3 Platelet-activating factor

Platelet-activating factor (PAF) is a potent inflammatory mediator that mimics many features of asthma, including eosinophil recruitment and activation and induction of AHR, plasma exudation, and mucus hypersecretion. The high level of lyso-PAF (metabolite of PAF) is analyzed in BALF of patients with allergic asthma [27].

2.4.4 Prostaglandin

Prostaglandins are generated from arachidonic acid by cyclooxygenase (COX) pathway. Increased concentration of PGF2, PGD2, and thromboxane B2 in bronchoalveolar (BAL) fluid of asthmatics is found. When inhaled, they cause bronchoconstriction [28] and increase airway responsiveness to spasmogen.

2.4.5 Proteases

Tryptase is a mast cell serine protease and plays a role in hemostasis, mucus secretion, and vascular permeability. Elevated levels of tryptase have been found in BAL fluid and sputum of asthmatic patients after allergen challenge [29]. Elevated levels of MMP-9 (metalloproteinase-9), a protease released by eosinophils and alveolar macrophages, are found in bronchoalveolar fluid from asthmatic patients [30].

2.4.6 Kinins

Kinins are vasoactive peptides secreted from kininogens by the action of kininogenase during the inflammatory response. Bradykinin is an important kinin that has many effects on airway functions mediated by direct activation of B2 receptors of airway smooth muscles. Bradykinin activates alveolar macrophages to release LTB_4 and PAF and activates nociceptive nerve fibers in the airways of asthmatic patients only which may mediate cough and chest tightness characteristic features of asthma [31] .

2.4.7 Cytokines

Cytokines are extracellular signaling proteins secreted by almost every cell under certain conditions and play a critical role in orchestrating all types of inflammatory response in asthma [32]. They act on target cells to cause a wide range of cellular functions like activation, proliferation, chemotaxis, immunomodulation, release of inflammatory mediators, growth and cell differentiation, and apoptosis. In contrast to acute and subacute inflammatory responses, cytokines play a dominant role in maintaining chronic inflammation in allergic diseases. The important cytokines in asthma are lymphokines secreted by T-lymphocytes: IL-1β, IL-3, IL-4, IL-5, IL-6, IL-9, IL-13, TNF-α, etc. where IL-3 is reported to be crucial for the survival of mast cells in tissues, but IL-4 plays an important role in switching B-lymphocytes to produce IgE and expression of VCAM-1 on endothelial cells. IL-5 plays a critical role in differentiation, survival, and priming of eosinophils, thus promoting eosinophilic inflammation, and present in BAL fluid during allergen-induced late-phase asthma [33]. Airway macrophages are important source of IL-1β, TNF- α, and IL-6 which act on epithelial cells to release GM-CSF, IL-8, and RANTES and amplify the inflammatory response leading to influx of secondary cells like eosinophils [34].

2.4.7.1 Proinflammatory cytokines

IL-9 and IL-13 are considered as proinflammatory cytokines. IL-9 is known to stimulate proliferation of activated T cells, enhancing IgE production from B cells, promoting proliferation and differentiation of mast cells, upregulating the α-chain of the FcεRI receptor, and inducing CC chemokine expression in lung epithelial cells contributing in allergen-induced airway changes. IL-13 is present in increased amounts in asthmatic airways and possesses biological activities similar to IL-4 [35]. Unlike IL-4 which is central to development of Th2 cells during primary sensitization, IL-13 release is more important during secondary antigen exposure [36].

Another group of proinflammatory cytokines are TNF-α that help in leukocyte recruitment through upregulation of adhesion molecules on vascular endothelial cells and induction of cytokine and chemokine synthesis airway hyper-responsiveness and pathogenesis of airway remodeling [37].

2.4.7.2 Immunomodulatory cytokines

IL-10, IL-12, IL-18, and interferon gamma (IFN-γ) are known as immunomodulatory cytokines. IL-10 is a pleiotropic cytokine that has the potential to downregulate both Th1- and Th2-driven inflammatory processes [38] and beneficial effect on airway remodeling [39]. IL-12 is released by antigen-presenting cells and is known to play an important role in Th1/Th2 differentiation during primary antigen presentation [40]. IL-18 is secreted by macrophages [41], and IFN-γ is reported to

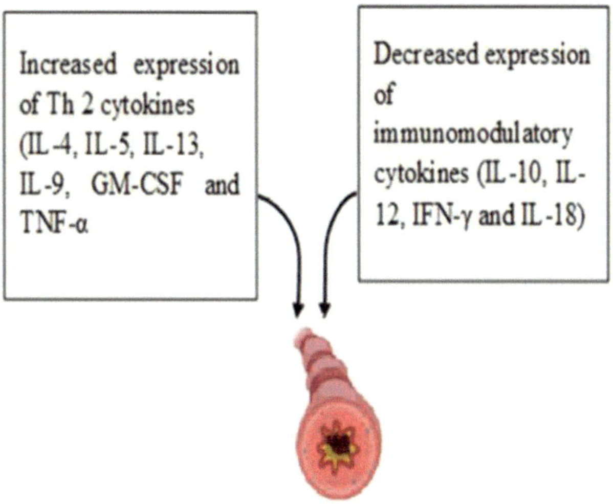

Figure 3.
Cytokines involved in the pathogenesis of bronchial asthma.

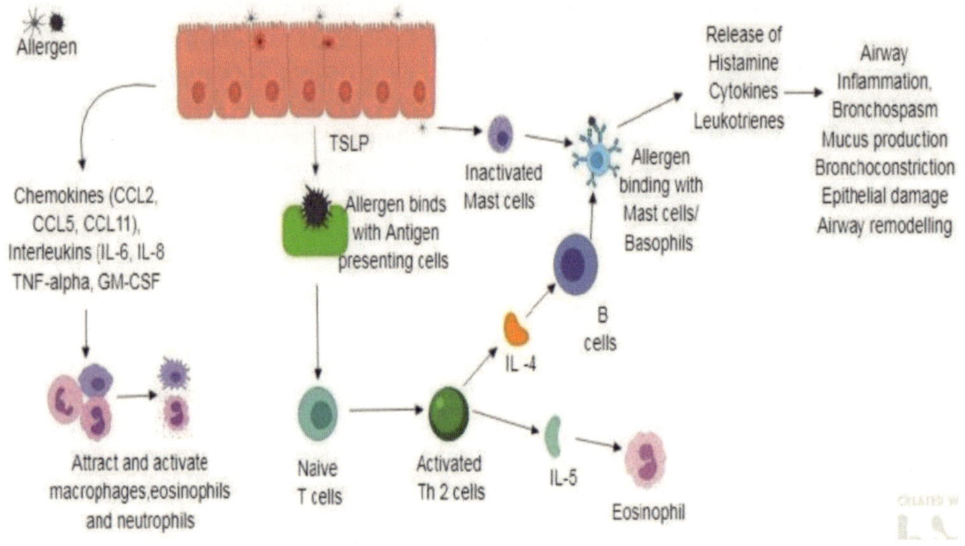

Figure 4.
Release of mediators after allergen exposure to airway epithelia.

prevent the development of antigen-induced airway eosinophilia and hyper-responsiveness [42]. IL-12 and IL-18 act synergistically for inducing IFN-γ and inhibiting IL-4-dependent IgE synthesis as well as inhibiting allergen-induced airway hyper-responsiveness [43]. Balance between Th1 and Th2 cells is thought to be determined by locally released cytokines, such as IL-12, which favor emergence of Th1 cells; contrary to this, IL-4 and IL-13 favor the growth of Th2 cells (**Figures 3** and **4**).

2.4.8 Chemokines

Chemokines are chemotactic cytokines responsible for recruitment of inflammatory cells in the airways. Chemokines have been categorized into two main groups, (a) CXC (α-type) and CC (β-type) chemokines, and exert their effects through G-protein-coupled chemokine receptors (CCR) [44]. Exacerbation of asthma leads to the synthesis and release of a number of chemokines. Increased expression of eotaxin, eotaxin-2, MCP-3, MCP-4, and CCR3 in the airways of asthmatic patients is found, and this can be correlated to increased AHR [45].

2.4.9 Tachykinins

Tachykinins are neuropeptides derived from preprotachykinins (PPTs). They are released by sensory nerves of airways and stimulate mucus secretion, plasma exudation, neural activation, bronchoconstriction, and structural changes. These peptides activate macrophages and monocytes to release inflammatory cytokines, IL-6 [46]. Higher concentration of a tachykinin, substance-P (SP), has been found in BALF of asthmatic lungs [47].

2.4.10 Endothelins

Endothelins are peptide mediators secreted via endothelin-converting enzyme (ECE) through mRNA present in airway epithelial cells and regulated by a number of proinflammatory cytokines in asthma. The biological effects of endothelins are mediated by two receptors: ET_A and ET_B. Endothelins are potent bronchoconstrictors and induce airway smooth muscle cell proliferation and fibrosis and play an important role in chronic inflammation of asthmatic airways [48]. After the allergen challenge, endothelins (ETs) are secreted de novo. Higher levels of endothelin-1 are found in the sputum of asthmatic patients [49].

2.4.11 Neural mediators

Several nonadrenergic-noncholinergic (NANC) nerves and neuropeptides have been identified in the respiratory tract. Airway nerves may also release neurotransmitters that have inflammatory effects such as substance P (SP), neurokinin A, and calcitonin gene-related peptide, may be released from sensitized inflammatory nerves in the airways, and perpetuate the ongoing inflammatory response. Thus, chronic asthma may be associated with increased neurogenic inflammation, which may provide a mechanism for prolonging the inflammatory response even in the absence of initiating inflammatory stimuli.

2.5 Antibodies

Antibodies are protein molecules released by immune system in response to foreign bodies, allergens. Five classes of antibodies, namely, IgM, IgG, IgA, IgD, and IgE [48], are known. Of these IgE is the predominant antibody in asthma in humans. IgE is the antibody responsible for all types of allergic reaction and pathogenesis of allergic asthma and development of inflammation in the human body. Elevated levels of IgE are found in bronchial asthma. Monoclonal antibodies against IgE have shown the reduction of IgE and associated asthma symptoms in asthmatics [50].

2.6 Oxidative stress

The increased level of oxidative stress found in airways of people with allergic asthma activates circulatory inflammatory cells, such as macrophages and eosinophils. Activated inflammatory cells produce more number of reactive oxygen species causing Increased concentrations of 8-isoprostane (a product of oxidized arachidonic acid) [51] and ethane (a product of oxidative lipid peroxidation) in exhaled breath of asthmatic patients [52]. Increased oxidative stress can be related to disease severity and may amplify the inflammatory response and reduce responsiveness to corticosteroids, particularly in severe disease and during exacerbations. Mechanism underlying the role of oxidative stress in asthma severity may be due to reaction of superoxide anions with nitric oxide (NO) forming reactive radical peroxynitrites that may modify several target proteins.

2.7 Nitric oxide (NO)

Measurement of the level of NO in exhaled air of asthmatic patients is increasingly being used as a noninvasive way of monitoring the inflammatory process [53]. NO is produced by NO synthase, but in epithelial cells of asthmatic patients, the enzyme inducible of NO synthase (iNOS) is present. Recent studies report the higher level of NO in the exhaled air of patients with asthma than the level of NO in the exhaled air of normal subjects. The combination of increased oxidative stress and NO may lead to the formation of the potent radical peroxynitrite that may result in nitrosylation of proteins in the airways [54]. Since NO is a potent vasodilator, this may increase plasma exudation in airways, and it may also amplify the Th2-mediated response.

3. Airway remodeling

The acute and chronic allergic inflammatory responses in asthmatic lungs result in epithelial shedding, goblet cell hyperplasia, basal membrane thickening, subepithelial fibrosis in peribronchial interstitial tissue, hyperplasia of airway smooth muscle cells, angiogenesis, and dysfunctioning of bronchial blood vessels [55]. These changes contribute to alteration in lung anatomy termed as airway remodeling and are represented by increased thickness of the basement membrane and increased volume of airway smooth muscle associated with increases in growth factors, including TGF-β_1 and platelet-derived growth factor, in Th2-driven models of asthma [56–58]. Overexpression of Th2 interleukins, especially IL-4, IL-5, and IL-13, is known to produce demonstrative changes in asthmatic airways. Increased expression of IL-13 causes subepithelial fibrosis, mucus metaplasia, and infiltration of eosinophils and macrophages, whereas increased expression of IL-4 and IL-5 induced airway eosinophilia, mucus metaplasia, and subepithelial fibrosis.

4. Conclusion

Complex interactions among various bioactive mediators in asthmatic lungs make it a complex disease and therefore need a more detailed research studies to discern its complete physiology.

Acknowledgements

The author is thankful to Jamia Hamdard for providing guidance in this research work.

Conflict of interest

The author declares no conflict of interest.

Author details

Poonam Arora* and S.H. Ansari
Jamia Hamdard, New Delhi, India

*Address all correspondence to: poonamarora96@gmail.com

References

[1] Blease K, Lukacs NW, Hogaboam CM, Kunkel SL. Chemokines and their role in airway hyper-reactivity. Respiratory Research. 2000;**1**:54-61

[2] Meagher LC, Cousin JM, Seckl JR, Haslett C. Opposing effects of glucocorticoids on the rate of apoptosis in neutrophilic and eosinophilic granulocytes. Journal of Immunology. 1996;**156**:4422-4428

[3] Wenzel S, Ford L, Pearlman D, Spector S, Sher L, Skobieranda F. Dupilumab in persistent asthma with elevated eosinophil levels. The New England Journal of Medicine. 2013;**368**:2455-2466

[4] Jatakanon A, Uasaf C, Maziak W, Lim S, Chung KF, Barnes PJ. Neutrophilic inflammation in severe persistent asthma. American Journal of Respiratory and Critical Care Medicine. 1999;**160**:1532-1539

[5] Sur S, Crotly TB, Kephart GM. Sudden-onset fatal asthma: A distinct entity with few eosinophils and relatively more neutrophils in the airway submucosal. The American Review of Respiratory Disease. 1993;**148**:713-719

[6] Lee TH, Lane SJ. The role of macrophages in the mechanisms of airway inflammation in asthma. The American Review of Respiratory Disease. 1992;**145**:S27-S30

[7] Poulter LW, Burke CM. Macrophages and allergic lung disease. Immunobiology. 1996;**195**:574-587

[8] Spiteri MA, Knight RA, Jeremy JY, Barnes PJ, Chung KF. Alveolar macrophage-induced suppression of peripheral blood mononuclear cell responsiveness is reversed by in vitro allergen exposure in bronchial asthma. The European Respiratory Journal. 1994;7:1431-1438

[9] Holt PG, McMenamin C. Defence against allergic sensitization in the healthy lung: The role of inhalation tolerance. Clinical and Experimental Allergy. 1989;**19**:255-262

[10] Carroll M, Mutavdzic S, James AL. Distribution and degranulation of airway mast cell in normal and asthmatics subjects. European Respiratory Journal. 2002;**19**:1-7

[11] Abul K, Abbas MD. Disease of immunity. In: Robbins and Cotran Pathologic Basis of Disease. 7th ed. Philadelphia, Pennsylvania: Elsevier Saunders; 2005. pp. 194-268

[12] Barnes PJ. Pathophysiology of allergic inflammation. Immunological Reviews. 2011;**242**:31-50

[13] Cosmi L, Liotta F, Maggi E, Romagnani S, Annunziato F. Th17 cells: New players in asthma pathogenesis. Allergy. 2011;**66**:989-998

[14] Lloyd CM, Saglani S. T cells in asthma: Influences of genetics, environment, and T-cell plasticity. Journal of Allergy and Clinical Immunology. 2013;**131**:1267-1274

[15] Bacharier LB, Jabara H, Geha RS. Molecular mechanisms of immunoglobulin E regulation. International Archives of Allergy and Immunology. 1998;**115**:257-269

[16] Elemam NM, Hannawi S, Maghazachi AA. Innate lymphoid cells (ILCs) as mediators of inflammation, release of cytokines and lytic molecules. Toxins. 2017;**9**:398

[17] Vivier E, Artis D, Colonna M, Diefenbach A, Di Santo JP, Eberl G, et al. Innate lymphoid cells: 10 years on. Cell. 2018;**174**(5):1054-1066

[18] Saenz SA, Siracusa MC, Perrigoue JG, Spencer SP, Urban JF Jr, Tocker

JE, et al. IL25 elicits a multipotent progenitor cell population that promotes T(H)2 cytokine responses. Nature. 2010;**464**:1362-1366

[19] Lambrecht BN, Hammad H. The airway epithelium in asthma. Nature Medicine. 2012;**18**:684-692

[20] Salazar F, Ghaemmaghami AM. Allergen recognition by innate immune cells: Critical role of dendritic and epithelial cells. Frontiers in Immunology. 2013;**4**:356

[21] Maazi H, Lam J, Lombardi V, Akbari O. Role of plasmacytoid dendritic cell subsets in allergic asthma. Allergy. 2013;**68**:695-701

[22] Walzog B, Gaehtgens P. Adhesion molecules: The path to a new understanding of acute inflammation. News in Physiological Sciences. 2000;**15**:107-113

[23] McAdam AJ, Chang TT, Lumelsky AE, Greenfield EA, Boussiotis VA, Duke-Cohan JS, et al. Mouse inducible costimulatory molecule (ICOS) expression is enhanced by CD28 costimulation and regulates differentiation of CD-4- T cells. Journal of Immunology. 2000;**165**:5035-5040

[24] Gonzalo JA, Tian J, Delaney T, Corcoran J, Rottman JB, Lora J, et al. ICOS is critical for T helper cell-mediated lung mucosal inflammatory responses. Nature Immunology. 2001;**2**:597-604

[25] Raible DG, Lenahan T, Fayvilevich Y, Kosinski R, Schulman ES. zPharmacological characterization of a novel histamine receptor on human eosinophil. American Journal of Respiratory and Critical Care Medicine. 1994;**149**:1506-1511

[26] Drazen JM, Israel E, O'Byrne PM. Treatment of asthma with drugs modifying the leukotriene pathway. The New England Journal of Medicine. 1999;**340**:197-206

[27] Tsukioka K, Matsuzaki M, Nakamata M, Kayahara H, Nakagawa T. Increased plasma level of platelet-activating factor (PAF) and decreased serum PAF acetylhydrolase (PAFAH) activity in adults with bronchial asthma. Journal of Investigational Allergology and Clinical Immunology. 1996;**6**:22-29

[28] Saroea HG, Inman MD, O'Byene PM. U46619 induced bronchoconstriction in asthmatic subjects is mediated by acetylcholine release. American Journal of Respiratory and Critical Care Medicine. 1995;**151**:321-324

[29] Louis R, Shule J, Biagi S, Stanciu L, Marrelli F, Tennor H, et al. Cell infiltration, ICAM-1 expression and eosinophil chemotactic activity in asthmatic sputum. American Journal of Respiratory and Critical Care Medicine. 1997;**155**:466-472

[30] Mautino G, Oliver N, Chanez P, Bousquet J, Capony F. Increased release of matrix metalloproteinease-9 in bronchoalveolar lavage fluid and by alveolar macrophages of asthmatics. American Journal of Respiratory Cell and Molecular Biology. 1997;**17**:583-591

[31] Bhoola KD, Figeroa CD, Worthy K. Bioregulation of kinins: Kallikerins, kiinogenins and kininases. Pharmacological Reviews. 1992;**44**:1-80

[32] Chung KF, Barnes PJ. Cytokines in asthma. Thorax. 1999;**54**:825-857

[33] Kita O, Weiler D, Sur S. IL-5 is the predominant eosinophil-active cytokine in the antigen-induced pulmonary late-phase reaction. The American Review of Respiratory Disease. 1993;**147**:901-907

[34] Peters-Golden M. The alveolar macrophages: The forgotten cell in asthma. American Journal of

Respiratory Cell and Molecular Biology. 2004;**31**(1):3-7

[35] Naseer T, Minshall EM, Leung DY. Expression of IL-12 and IL-13 mRNA in asthma and their modulation in response to steroid therapy. American Journal of Respiratory and Critical Care Medicine. 1997;**155**:845-851

[36] De-Vries JE. The role of IL-13 and its receptor in allergy and inflammatory responses. The Journal of Allergy and Clinical Immunology. 1998;**102**:165-169

[37] Hirata N, Kohrogi H, Iwagoe H, et al. Allergen exposure induces the expression of endothelial adhesion molecules in passively sensitized human bronchus: Time course and the role of cytokines. American Journal of Respiratory Cell and Molecular Biology. 1998;**18**:12-20

[38] Koulis A, Robinson DS. The anti-inflammatory effects of interleukin-10 in allergic disease. Clinical and Experimental Allergy. 2000;**30**:747-750

[39] Selzman CH, McIntyre RC, Shames BD, Whitehill TA, Banerjee A, Harken AH. Interleukin-10 inhibits human vascular smooth muscle proliferation. Journal of Molecular and Cellular Cardiology. 1998;**30**:889-896

[40] Rissoan MC, Soumelis V, Kadowaki NJ. Reciprocal control of T helper cell and dendritic cell differentiation. Science. 1999;**283**:1183-1186

[41] Okamura H, Tsutsi H, Komatsu T. Cloning of a new cytokine that induces IFN-gamma production by T cells. Nature. 1995;**378**:88-91

[42] Lack G, Bradley KL, Hamelmann E. Nebulized IFN-gamma inhibits the development of secondary allergic responses in mice. Journal of Immunology. 1996;**157**:1432-1439

[43] Hofstra CL, Van Ark I, Hofman G, Kool M, Nijkamp FP, Van Oosterhout AJ. Prevention of Th2-like cell responses by co-administration of IL-12 and IL-18 is associated with inhibition of antigen-induced airway hyper-responsiveness, eosinophilia, and serum IgE levels. Journal of Immunology. 1998;**161**:5054-5060

[44] Barnes PJ. Intrinsic asthma: Not so different from allergic asthma but driven by superantigens? Clinical and Experimental Allergy. 2009;**39**:1145-1151

[45] Ying S, Meng Q, Zeibecoglou K, et al. Eosinophil chemotactic chemokines (eotaxin, eotaxin-2, RANTES, monocyte chemoattractant protein-3 (MCP-3), and MCP-4), and C-C chemokine receptor 3 expression in bronchial biopsies from atopic and nonatopic (intrinsic) asthmatics. Journal of Immunology. 1999;**163**:6321-6329

[46] Brunelleschi S, Vanni L, Ledda F, Giotti A, Maggi CA, Fantozzi R. Tachykinins activate guinea pig alveolar macrophages: Involvement of NK-2 and NK1 receptors. British Journal of Pharmacology. 1990;**100**:417-420

[47] Nieber K, Baumgarten CR, Rathsack R, Furkert J, Oehame P, Kunkel G. Substance P and b endorphin-like immunoreactivity in lavage fluids of subjects with and without asthma. The Journal of Allergy and Clinical Immunology. 1992;**90**:646-652

[48] Goldie RG, Henry PJ. Endothelins and asthma. Life Sciences. 1999;**65**:1-15

[49] Redington AE, Springall DR, Ghatei MA. Airway endothelin levels in asthma: Influence of endobronchial allergen challenge and maintenance corticosteroid therapy. The European Respiratory Journal. 1997;**10**:1026-1032

[50] Busse WW, Holgate ST, Simons FER, Yunginger JW, editors. Middleton's

Allergy Principles and Practce. 6th ed. Philadelphia: Molsby; 2003. pp. 887-913

[51] Montuschi P, Ciabattoni G, Corradi M, et al. Increased 8-Isoprostane, a marker of oxidative stress, in exhaled condensates of asthmatic patients. American Journal of Respiratory and Critical Care Medicine. 1999;**160**:216-220

[52] Paredi P, Kharitonov SA, Barnes PJ. Elevation of exhaled ethane concentration in asthma. American Journal of Respiratory and Critical Care Medicine. 2000;**162**:1450-1454

[53] Kharitonov SA, Barnes PJ. Clinical aspects of exhaled nitric oxide. The European Respiratory Journal. 2000;**16**:781-792

[54] Saleh D, Ernst P, Lim S, Barnes PJ, Giaid A. Increased formation of the potent oxidant peroxynitrite in the airways of asthmatic patients is associated with induction of nitric oxide synthase: Effect of inhaled glucocorticoid. The FASEB Journal. 1998;**12**:929-937

[55] Fehrenbach H, Wagner C, Wegmann M. Airway remodeling in asthma: What really matters. Cell and Tissue Research. 2017;**367**(3):551-569

[56] Mason RJ, Murray JF, Broaddus VC, Nadel JA, editors. Murray and Nadel's Textbook of Respiratory Medicine. 4th ed. Philadelphia: Saunders/Elseviers Publication; 2005. pp. 51-86

[57] Holgate ST. Epithelium dysfunction in asthma. The Journal of Allergy and Clinical Immunology. 2007;**120**(6):1233-1244

[58] Jeffery PK. Remodeling in asthma and chronic obstructive lung disease. American Journal of Respiratory and Critical Care Medicine. 2001;**164**:S28-S38

Chapter 8

Pathogenic Roles of MicroRNA in the Development of Asthma

Xiaoyan Dong and Nanbert Zhong

Abstract

Asthma is a common and chronic inflammatory disease. Pathogenic mechanism underlying asthma is complicated. The inflammatory reactions in asthma have been recognized to involve mast cells, eosinophils, lymphocytes (T cells, B cells), macrophages, and dendritic cells. MicroRNA (miRNA, miR) is a group of small noncoding RNAs with 21–25 nucleotides (nt) in length, which impact biologic responses through the regulation of mRNA transcription and/or translation. MicroRNAs are related to developmental processes of many immunologic diseases. Most studies showed that regulation of miRNAs to their targeting genes appears to play an important role in the development of asthma. This chapter has discussed altered expression of miRNAs in cells and tissues from patients with asthma, in order to better understand the mechanics of pathogenesis of asthma. In addition, the regulation of miRNAs as a novel therapeutic approach will require a deeper understanding of their function and mechanism of action.

Keywords: microRNA asthma, inflammation reaction

1. Introduction

Pediatric asthma is a global problem. In the last decade, its incidence has highly increased, particular growing by 10% in China [1]. Etiologically, asthma attack, due to gene-environmental interactions, can also be induced by allergy factors, including air pollution, pollen, fungi and dust mites, food, and so on [2]. As a chronic inflammatory disease and a polygenic hereditary disease, the mechanism of asthma is not clearly understood until now. The adaptive and innate immune system with the involvement of mast cells, eosinophils, lymphocytes (T cells, B cells), macrophages, and dendritic cells, even epithelial cells and structure cells, contributed to the inflammation reaction of asthma [3–5]. Moreover, change in the secretion of IgE and cytokines, including gamma-interferon (γ-IFN) and tumor necrosis factor (TNF-α), is important in asthma attacks [6–8]. As an immune regulator, microRNA (miRNA or miR) regulates on target gene mRNA and plays an important role in the development and pathogenesis of asthma.

MicroRNAs are a group of small nonprotein-coding RNAs that are 21–25 nucleotides in length. They act as transcriptional regulators involved in many complex human disorders and in biological processes including cell proliferation and apoptosis [9, 10]. Childhood asthma susceptibility is associated with mutations in specific gene mRNA and/or their specific miRNA. For example, HLA-G has been identified as an asthma susceptibility gene [11], which was found to be the target gene of miR-148a, miR-148b, and miR-152. Further support for the theory that miRNA changes may be the cause of childhood asthma. The specific genotype of children with asthma was related to the significant difference in allele polymorphism (SNP) of rs2910164G/C and rs2292832C/T of pre-miRNA [12]. It showed that miR-223 was involved in the maturation and function of neutrophil differentiation [13]. miR-27b-3p, miR-513a-5p, and miR-22-3p were also indicated to have influenced dust mite-induced asthma by regulating its target gene [14, 15]. In a murine model of acute and chronic asthma study, abnormal expression of miRNAs including miR-146b, miR-223, miR-29b, miR-29c, miR-483, miR-5745p, miR-672, and miR-690 in asthma was

miRNA	Inflammatory response	Reaction and cell differentiate	Reference
miRNA-223	Immune inflammatory response	Neutrophils mature and differentiate	[13]
miRNA-146, miRNA-146a	Asthma, innate immune responses	Airway epithelium, NF-kappaB pathway	[17, 18]
miRNA-147	Immune inflammatory response	TLR signaling pathway	[19]
miRNA-145	Asthma	Comparable to glucocorticoid treatment	[20]
miRNA-155	Immune inflammatory response, asthma	TLR signaling pathway, regulation of allergic inflammation, macrophage inflammatory response, Th2 priming of dendritic cells	[21–24]
miRNA-21	Immune inflammatory response, asthma	TLR signaling pathway, NF-kB, IL-12p35 polarization	[25–27]
miRNA-124	Allergy inflammation	M2 phenotype of monocytic cells	[28]
miRNA-148a, miR-148b, and miR-152	Asthma	HLA-G	[11, 29]
miRNA-126	Asthma	Th2 response, airway hyperresponse	[30]
let-7	Asthma	Il-13, regulation of allergic inflammation	[31–33]
miRNA-221	Asthma	Mast cell activity regulates the production of cytokines	[34, 35]
miRNA-9	Asthma	Regulates steroid-resistant airway hyperresponsiveness	[36]
miRNA-672, miRNA-143	Asthma	Expression of metalloproteinase	[37]
miR-19a	Asthma	Enhances proliferation of bronchial epithelial cells by targeting TGFbetaR2 gene	[38]
miRNA-203	Asthma	Negatively regulates c-Abl, ERK1/2 phosphorylation, and proliferation in smooth muscle cells	[39]
miRNA-133, miR-133a	Asthma	Upregulation of Rhoa in bronchial smooth muscle cells	[40]
miR-192	Asthma	Decreased expression in peripheral blood of asthmatic individuals undergoing an allergen inhalation challenge	[41]

Table 1.
The relationship of miRNA and inflammation response.

detected [16]. It was found that miRNA plays an important role in regulating immune pathway(s). A lot of studies have focused on the relationship between miRNA and asthma during decades, which involved not only in inflammation cells and cytokines but also in the treatment of glucocorticoids (**Table 1**). In this chapter, we discuss the relationship of miRNAs to their targeted mRNA(s) involved in the inflammation cell in asthma, in order to review the pathogenic mechanism of asthma.

2. miRNA in T cell and B cell

T cell and B cell play an important role in immune mechanism, especially innate and adaptive immunity, of asthma. As an immune regulator, miRNA influences on these two cells and regulates their proliferation and function. Many studies have been focused on the regulation of miRNA to T cell and B cell in order to clear the mechanism of asthma.

2.1 T cell, follicular helper T cells (TFH cells), and Th17

T follicular helper (Tfh) cells are essential for the formation of germinal centers (GCs). As a subset of CD4+, it mediates GC formation and maintenance and provides help to antigen-specific B cells during infection and vaccination. Th17 cells have also been implicated in the pathogenesis of several autoimmune and inflammatory diseases [42–44]. Th17 cells also mediate immune responses that are involved in maintaining epithelial barrier integrity, and it has been widely suggested that some cases of asthma may be caused by dysregulated Th17 responses [44, 45]. MiRNA also regulates the differentiation and function of these cells.

It was found that the miR-17-92 cluster's increasing role in regulating the immune system is involved in innate and adaptive immunity, including B cells and subsets of T cells such as Th1, Th2, T follicular helper cells, regulatory T cells, monocytes/macrophages, NK cells, and dendritic cells [46]. Moreover, the study found that the miR-17 approximately 92 cluster is a critical regulator of T cell-dependent antibody responses and follicular helper T cells' (TFH cells) differentiation [47].

We knew that the relationship of miRNA and its target gene mRNA is not a one-to-one correspondence. Target gene mRNA could be regulated by many miRNAs, or one miRNA could regulate a number of mRNAs. A study showed that some miRNAs with strong probability may induce miR-27b, miR-27a, miR-30c, miR-1, and miR-141 or inhibit miR-20b, miR-93, miR-20a, miR-152, miR-21, and miR-106a in Th17 differentiation by targeting negative or positive regulators of Th17 differentiation, respectively [48]. In a regulatory network model of murine T helper cell differentiation, the miR-212~132 and miR-182~183 clusters were significantly upregulated, and the overall miR-106~363 cluster was downregulated, which predicted to affect Th17 cell differentiation. In vitro, when miR-18b, miR-106a, and miR-363-3p were transfected into primary murine Cd4(+) lymphocytes, the expression of retinoid-related orphan receptor c (Rorc), Rora, IL17a, and IL17f and abolished secretion of Th17-mediated interleukin-17a (IL17a) have declined [49].

In addition, miR-18a directly targeted Smad4, Hif1a, and Rora in the Th17 cell gene expression program. All of these reveal that activating signals influence the outcome of Th cell differentiation via differential regulation of mature microRNAs within a common cluster [50]. miR-18a was the most dynamically upregulated microRNA of the miR-17-92 cluster during Th17 cell differentiation. Based on which, the involvement of miR-18a in the regulation of T-cell differentiation was demonstrated.

miR-155, as an important regulator in asthma, was involved in many pathways in allergy disease in **Table 1**. It was shown that the function in macrophage inflammatory response [23] is differentially expressed in allergic T cells exposed to DM extract compared to in nonallergic cells. The level of miR-155 expression was positively associated with the expression of the TH2 cytokines IL-5 and IL-13. When miR-155 was inhibited by glucocorticoids in Jurkat T cells, then the production of these cytokines were inhibited [51].

Several differentially expressed miRNAs in asthma, such as miRNA-34/449, let-7, miRNA-19, miRNA-21, and miRNA-455, were identified in various cell types and tissues including epithelial cells, T cells, type 2 innate lymphoid cells, lung tissues, and smooth muscles. These miRNAs are involved in epithelial differentiation, mucus production, airway remodeling, and inflammation as well [52]. miR-146a has been shown to modulate T-cell immunity as well as enhance class switch and secretion of IgE in B cells by upregulating 14-3-3 sigma expression [53].

2.2 miRNA regulates B cell

B cells play a critical role in immune responses, but the regulation of microRNAs to B-cell proliferation and function was partially understood. Not only miR-17-92 cluster was involved in B cell [46], but miR-146a also enhances class switch and secretion of IgE in B cells [53]. As an important immune regulatory cell, thrombospondin 1 (TSP1)-producing B cells were regulated by miRNAs as well. miR-98 can suppress the expression of TSP1 in the peripheral B cells of patients with allergic asthma [54]. Further study revealed that overexpression of miR-29b in human B cells precipitated a reduction in overall AID protein whose activity affected the function of class-switch recombination (CSR) and then results in corresponding diminution in CSR to IgE [55].

3. miRNA and mast cell

It is essential that mast cells have major effector and immune regulatory functions in IgE-associated allergic diseases or in innate and adaptive immune responses. But their mechanism was not clear yet. miRNAs provide an additional layer in the regulation of gene expression acting as repressors with several targets at the posttranscriptional level. Several studies showed that miRNA expression patterns during differentiation and activation of mast cells. The expression of many miRNAs changes following IgE-FcepsilonRI cross-linking in activated mast cells. Upregulated expression of miR-221 promotes IgE-mediated activation of mast cell degranulation by PI3K/Akt/PLCgamma/Ca^{2+} signaling pathway, in a non-NF-kappaB-dependent manner [56]. Downregulation of miR-223 promotes degranulation *via* the PI3K/Akt pathway by targeting IGF-1R in mast cells [57]. In cockroach allergen model of asthma, when miRNA-33b was overexpressed, mast cell degranulation was inhibited through suppression of the calcium release and IgE-FcepsilonRI pathway [58]. In line with this, neutralization of miR-132 by anti-miR inhibitor leads to sustained production of HB-EGF protein in activated mast cells [59].

Cytokine is also related to miRNA and mast cells in inflammation response of asthma. The treatment of IL-10 has been shown to suppress TNF production in mast cells. IL-10 effects are dependent on Stat3 activation, eliciting miR-155 expression, with a resulting loss of suppressor of cytokine signaling-1 [60]. miR-221, which was overexpressed in a murine asthma model, stimulated IL-4 secretion in mast cells through a pathway involving PTEN, p38, and NF-kappaB [61]. miR-223 reduces IL-6 secretion in mast cells by inhibiting the IGF1R/PI3K signaling pathway [62]. Mex-3B, an antisense oligonucleotide targeting, directly upregulates IL-33 expression by inhibiting miR-487b-3p-mediated repression of IL-33 [63].

4. miRNA and dendritic cells

Dendritic cells (DCs) are the professional antigen-presenting cells (APCs) in the lung. They are found to be crucial in the induction and maintenance of allergic asthma by cross-linking innate and adaptive immune responses. After transfection with miR-23b reagents, DCs were evaluated for endocytic ability, surface marker expression, cytokine secretion, and CD4+ T-cell differentiation. The study proved that miR-23b is capable of inducing tolerogenic DC activity and Treg responses in vitro through the inhibition of the Notch1 and NF-kappaB signaling pathways; thus, miR-23b might represent a therapeutic target for the management of allergic diseases [64].

miR-155 has been shown to be a crucial regulator of the immune system mentioned above. Not only miR-155 can influence on T cell function but also regulate the activity of DCs. Deficiency of miR-155 on DCs was also associated with impaired purinergic receptor signaling and alleviates AAI by diminishing Th2 priming capacity and ATP-/P2R-induced activation of DCs in mice [24].

5. miRNA and inflammatory phenotype (neutrophilic asthma and eosinophilic asthma)

Asthma may be classified according to severity and inflammatory phenotype and is likely to be distinguished by specific microRNA (miRNA) expression profiles. The study of miRNA expression in sputum supernatants with the inflammatory cells in severe asthma was taken out. Expression of miR-629-3p, miR-223-3p, and miR-142-3p was significantly upregulated in the sputum of patients with severe asthma compared with that in healthy control subjects and was highest in patients with neutrophilic asthma. It suggested that these miRNAs are related to asthma inflammatory phenotype [65].

Single-nucleotide polymorphisms (SNPs) in miRNAs could affect their efficiency in binding to messenger RNAs (mRNAs), which was taken little into account before. In a study in Korean population, it showed that the CT/CC genotype of miR-196a2 at locus rs11614913 was associated with eosinophilic asthma and a higher sputum eosinophil count than the TT genotype. The CG/GG genotype at rs2910164 of miR-146a had a hyperresponsiveness in airway compared with the CC genotype. The AG/GG genotype at rs3746444 of miR-499 manifested higher predicted values of forced expiratory volume in 1 s (%FEV1) than the AA genotype [66].

A study about evaluating clinical potential of plasma miR-21 and miR-146a involved in T helper cell differentiation in childhood asthma found that the levels of miR-21 and miR-146a were not only positively correlated with eosinophil percentage but also associated with FEV1. miR-21 and miR-146a are upregulated in asthmatic children. miR-21 and miR-146a play a role in eosinophilic endotypic classification of asthma [67]. Moreover, its data show that miR-185-5p profile in eosinophils can be used as asthma diagnosis biomarker in serum and that this profile is able to rank asthma severity [68].

6. miRNA and macrophage

Monocytes and macrophages are important roles of the immune system, which possess pleiotropic effector and immunoregulatory functions. Classical activation (M1) and alternative activation (M2) of macrophages are necessary in the function. M1 polarization of macrophages results in the production of proinflammatory cytokines and antimicrobial and tumoricidal activity, whereas M2 polarization of macrophages is related to immunosuppression, tumorigenesis, wound repair, and elimination of parasites [69]. It also reveals that miRNAs were involved in M macrophages' activity. miR-511 is increased in macrophages following IL-4 and IL-13 stimulation and decreased in M1 macrophages both in vitro and in vivo [70]. Particularly, miR-9, miR-127, miR-155, and miR-125b have been shown to promote M1 polarization, while miR-124, miR-223, miR-34a, let-7c, miR-132, miR-146a, and miR-125a-5p may induce M2 polarization in macrophages by targeting various transcription factors and adaptor proteins. Differentiation of monocytes to macrophages is inhibited by miR-24, miR-30b, miR-142-3p, and miR-199a-5p. MiR-155 and miR-142-3p inhibit macrophage proliferation, compared to let-7a. Interestingly, miR-155 has both pro- and antiapoptotic roles, whereas miR-21 and let-7e negatively regulate macrophage apoptosis [69, 71, 72]. These data revealed that the function of miRNAs in modulating macrophage polarization may have potential way in the treatment of inflammation-related diseases.

On the other hand, studying the development of allergy disease in maternal pregnancy revealed that the embryonic development is highly sensitive to xenobiotic toxicity. If exposed to environmental toxins in utero, it affects physiological responses of the progeny. In the animal model, there was a lower expression of miR-130a and increased expression of miR-16 and miR-221 in the lungs of mice which were exposed to sidestream cigarette smoke (SS) or secondhand smoke exhibit. These miRNAs regulate HIF-1 alpha-regulated apoptotic, angiogenic, and immune pathways. This process will lead to increase incidence of allergic asthma (AA) and bronchopulmonary dysplasia (BPD) in the progenies [73].

Besides, the expression of miRNAs was different in fungal bioaerosols which are ubiquitous in the environment, and human exposure can result in a variety of health effects ranging from systemic, subcutaneous, and cutaneous infections to respiratory morbidity including allergy, asthma, and hypersensitivity pneumonitis. It was found that miRNAs were involved in the inflammatory stimuli exposure to fungal. In studies of exposures to fungi (such as *Aspergillus fumigatus*, *Candida albicans*, and *Cryptococcus neoformans*), it was revealed that several miRNAs that were shared between responses to these species including miR-125 a/miR-125 b, miR-132 [43], miR-146a, and miR-29a/miR-29b were also involved in macrophage polarization/activation, TLR-mediated signaling, natural killer cell function, C-leptin signaling, and inhibition of Th1 immune response, respectively [74]. On the other hand, miR-487b can suppress the levels of mRNA and protein for IL-33, which plays an important role in macrophage activation for innate host defense and proinflammatory responses during the differentiation of bone marrow-derived macrophages (BMDMs) [75].

In summary, miRNAs exert their effect by binding to complementary nucleotide sequences of the targeted messenger RNA, thus forming an RNA-induced silencing complex. miRNAs play important roles in many aspects of macrophage biology and thereby affect many biological and pathological conditions, like monocyte differentiation and development, macrophage polarization, infection, tumor growth, inflammatory activation, and so on [71, 72]. Numerous studies have demonstrated the important role of miRNA in the pathogenesis of childhood asthma, suggesting that miRNA plays a regulatory role between genes and the environment as well as allergic airway inflammation. The mechanism of miRNA activity involves a large number of miRNAs, which take mRNA with multiple functions as target genes and synergistically regulate multiple aspects of complex pathophysiological processes in childhood asthma. The role of miRNAs in inflammation cells is important in both innate and acquired immunity in which T cell, B cell, mast cells, macrophages, and dendritic cells are involved. The role of miRNAs in these cell types, miR-17-92 cluster, miR-221, miR-223, miR-146a, and miR-155, may be crucial

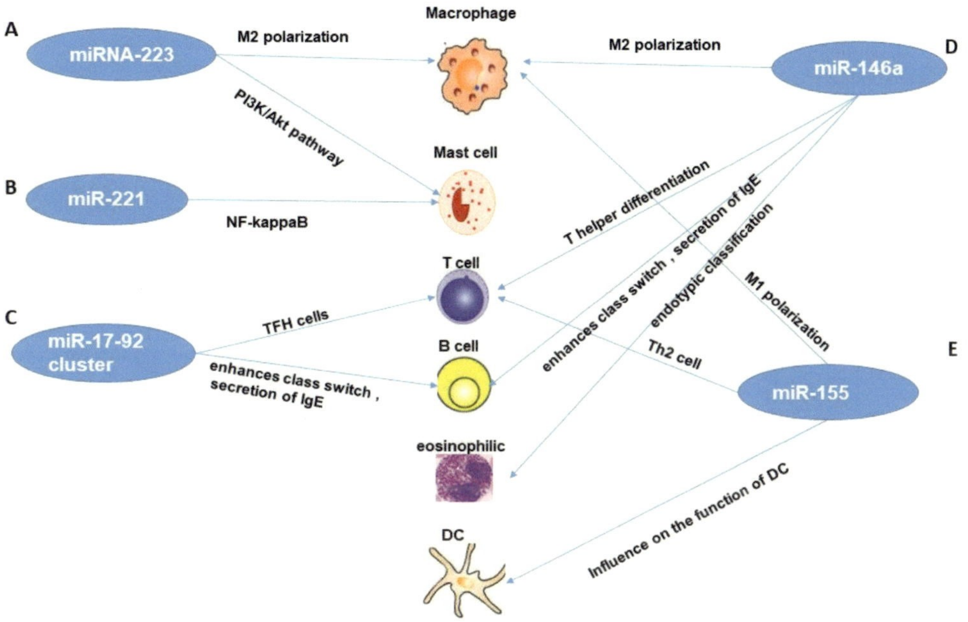

Figure 1.
miR-17-92 cluster, miR-221, miR-223, miR-146a, and miR-155 are associated with inflammation cells. (A) Downregulation of miR-223 promotes degranulation via the PI3K/Akt pathway by targeting IGF-1R and reduces IL-6 secretion in mast cells. It also induced M2 polarization. (B) miR-221 promoted IgE-mediated activation of mast cells degranulation by PI3K/Akt/PLCgamma/Ca^{2+} signaling pathway and stimulated IL-4 secretion in mast cells through a pathway involving PTEN, p38, and NF-kappaB. (C) miR-17~92 cluster as a critical regulator of T-cell-dependent antibody responses and follicular helper T cell (TFH cell) and Th17 differentiation. It enhances class switch and secretion of IgE in B cells. (D) miR-146 modulated T-cell immunity and enhanced class switch and secretion of IgE in B cells. miR-146a played a role in eosinophilic endotypic classification of asthma. It induced M2 polarization as well. (E) miR-155 was associated with Th2 cell and cytokine secretion. Deficiency of miR-155 on DCs was also related to impaired purinergic receptor signaling and alleviates AAI by diminishing Th2 priming capacity and ATP-/P2R-induced activation of DCs. It promoted M1 polarization.

(**Figure 1**). Depending on these roles of miRNAs in dendritic cells, mast cells, and macrophages, we speculate about possible future directions in the field [76]. It is likely variant miRNAs form a network in which these miRNAs may interact with each other and alter the expression of target genes in the inflammation process of pediatric asthma. On the other hand, it is envisaged that targeted manipulation of specific miRNAs could be developed as a new treatment for asthma. At present, our group has already had some result about the relationship of miRNA to target gene in dust mite-induced asthma. Depending on this review, further investigation should be pursued on the immune regulatory function of miRNA in children's asthma.

Acknowledgements

This study was supported by Shanghai Science and Science Commission International Cooperation Project (No. 18410721300) and Project on the cross project of Shanghai Jiaotong University (YG2017MS34).

Conflict of interest

There was no conflict of interest (economic, personal, scientific, healthcare, educational, religious, and social) interfering with the chapter.

Author details

Xiaoyan Dong[1] and Nanbert Zhong[2*]

1 Department of Pulmonary, Shanghai Children's Hospital, Shanghai Jiaotong University School of Medicine, Shanghai, China

2 New York State Institute for Basic Research in Developmental Disabilities, Staten Island, NY, USA

*Address all correspondence to: nanbert.zhong@opwdd.ny.gov

References

[1] The National Cooperative Group on Childhood Asthma, Institute of Environmental Health and Related Product Safety, Chinese Center for Disease Control and Prevention. Third nation wide survey of childhood asthma in urban areas of China. Chinese Journal of Pediatrics. 2013;**51**:729-740

[2] Rottier BL, Eber E, Hedlin G, Turner S, Wooler E, Mantzourani E, et al. Monitoring asthma in childhood: Management-related issues. European Respiratory Review. 2015;**24**:194-203

[3] Snijders D, Agostini S, Bertuola F, Panizzolo C, Baraldo S, Turato G, et al. Markers of eosinophilic and neutrophilic inflammation in bronchoalveolar lavage of asthmatic and atopic children. Allergy. 2010;**65**:978-985

[4] Larose MC, Chakir J, Archambault AS, Joubert P, Provost V, Laviolette M, et al. Correlation between CCL26 production by human bronchial epithelial cells and airway eosinophils: Involvement in patients with severe eosinophilic asthma. The Journal of Allergy and Clinical Immunology. Oct 2015;**136**(4):904-913

[5] Roth M, Zhao F, Zhong J, Lardinois D, Tamm M. Serum IgE induced airway smooth muscle cell remodeling is independent of allergens and is prevented by omalizumab. PLoS One. 2015;**10**:e0136549

[6] Chang YJ, DeKruyff RH, Umetsu DT. The role of type 2 innate lymphoid cells in asthma. Journal of Leukocyte Biology. 2013;**94**:933-940

[7] Sumino K, Tucker J, Shahab M, Jaffee KF, Visness CM, Gern JE, et al. Antiviral IFN-gamma responses of monocytes at birth predict respiratory tract illness in the first year of life. The Journal of Allergy and Clinical Immunology. 2012;**129**(1267-1273):e1261

[8] Choi JP, Kim YS, Kim OY, Kim YM, Jeon SG, Roh TY, et al. TNF-alpha is a key mediator in the development of Th2 cell response to inhaled allergens induced by a viral PAMP double-stranded RNA. Allergy. 2012;**67**:1138-1148

[9] Zhang B, Farwell MA. microRNAs: A new emerging class of players for disease diagnostics and gene therapy. Journal of Cellular and Molecular Medicine. 2008;**12**:3-21

[10] Pauley KM, Cha S, Chan EK. MicroRNA in autoimmunity and autoimmune diseases. Journal of Autoimmunity. 2009;**32**:189-194

[11] Tan Z, Randall G, Fan J, Camoretti-Mercado B, Brockman-Schneider R, Pan L, et al. Allele-specific targeting of microRNAs to HLA-G and risk of asthma. American Journal of Human Genetics. 2007;**81**:829-834

[12] Su XW, Yang Y, Lv ML, Li LJ, Dong W, Miao L, et al. Association between single-nucleotide polymorphisms in pre-miRNAs and the risk of asthma in a Chinese population. DNA and Cell Biology. 2011;**30**:919-923

[13] Johnnidis JB, Harris MH, Wheeler RT, Stehling-Sun S, Lam MH, Kirak O, et al. Regulation of progenitor cell proliferation and granulocyte function by microRNA-223. Nature. 2008;**451**:1125-1129

[14] Dong X, Xu M, Ren Z, Gu J, Lu M, Lu Q, et al. Regulation of CBL and ESR1 expression by microRNA-223p, 513a-5p and 625-5p may impact the pathogenesis of dust mite-induced pediatric asthma. International Journal of Molecular Medicine. 2016;**38**:446-456

[15] Dong X, Zhong N, Fang Y, Cai Q, Lu M, Lu Q. MicroRNA 27b-3p modulates SYK in pediatric asthma induced by

dust mites. Frontiers in Pediatrics. 22 Oct 2018;**6**:301. DOI: 10.3389/fped.2018.00301. eCollection 2018

[16] Garbacki N, Di Valentin E, Huynh-Thu VA, Geurts P, Irrthum A, Crahay C, et al. MicroRNAs profiling in murine models of acute and chronic asthma: A relationship with mRNAs targets. PLoS One. 2011;**6**:e16509

[17] Liu X, Nelson A, Wang X, Kanaji N, Kim M, Sato T, et al. MicroRNA-146a modulates human bronchial epithelial cell survival in response to the cytokine-induced apoptosis. Biochemical and Biophysical Research Communications. 2009;**380**:177-182

[18] Taganov KD, Boldin MP, Chang KJ, Baltimore D. NF-kappaB-dependent induction of microRNA miR-146, an inhibitor targeted to signaling proteins of innate immune responses. Proceedings of the National Academy of Sciences of the United States of America. 2006;**103**:12481-12486

[19] Liu G, Friggeri A, Yang Y, Park YJ, Tsuruta Y, Abraham E. miR-147, a microRNA that is induced upon Toll-like receptor stimulation, regulates murine macrophage inflammatory responses. Proceedings of the National Academy of Sciences of the United States of America. 2009;**106**:15819-15824

[20] Collison A, Mattes J, Plank M, Foster PS. Inhibition of house dust mite-induced allergic airways disease by antagonism of microRNA-145 is comparable to glucocorticoid treatment. The Journal of Allergy and Clinical Immunology. 2011;**128**(160-167):e164

[21] Tang B, Xiao B, Liu Z, Li N, Zhu ED, Li BS, et al. Identification of MyD88 as a novel target of miR-155, involved in negative regulation of *Helicobacter pylori*-induced inflammation. FEBS Letters. 2010;**584**:1481-1486

[22] Zhang YY, Zhong M, Zhang MY, Lv K. Expression and clinical significance of miR-155 in peripheral blood CD4(+);T cells of patients with allergic asthma. Chinese Journal of Cellular and Molecular Immunology. 2012;**28**:540-543

[23] O'Connell RM, Taganov KD, Boldin MP, Cheng G, Baltimore D. MicroRNA-155 is induced during the macrophage inflammatory response. Proceedings of the National Academy of Sciences of the United States of America. 2007;**104**:1604-1609

[24] Zech A, Ayata CK, Pankratz F, Meyer A, Baudiss K, Cicko S, et al. MicroRNA-155 modulates P2R signaling and Th2 priming of dendritic cells during allergic airway inflammation in mice. Allergy. 2015;**70**:1121-1129

[25] Lu TX, Munitz A, Rothenberg ME. MicroRNA-21 is up-regulated in allergic airway inflammation and regulates IL-12p35 expression. Journal of Immunology. 2009;**182**:4994-5002

[26] Sheedy FJ, Palsson-McDermott E, Hennessy EJ, Martin C, O'Leary JJ, Ruan Q, et al. Negative regulation of TLR4 via targeting of the proinflammatory tumor suppressor PDCD4 by the microRNA miR-21. Nature Immunology. 2010;**11**:141-147

[27] Sawant DV, Yao W, Wright Z, Sawyers C, Tepper RS, Gupta SK, et al. Serum microRNA-21 as a biomarker for allergic inflammatory disease in children. MicroRNA. 2015;**4**:36-40

[28] Veremeyko T, Siddiqui S, Sotnikov I, Yung A, Ponomarev ED. IL-4/IL-13-dependent and independent expression of miR-124 and its contribution to M2 phenotype of monocytic cells in normal conditions and during allergic inflammation. PLoS One. 2013;**8**:e81774

[29] Nicodemus-Johnson J, Laxman B, Stern RK, Sudi J, Tierney CN,

Norwick L, et al. Maternal asthma and microRNA regulation of soluble HLA-G in the airway. The Journal of Allergy and Clinical Immunology. 2013;**131**:1496-1503

[30] Mattes J, Collison A, Plank M, Phipps S, Foster PS. Antagonism of microRNA-126 suppresses the effector function of TH2 cells and the development of allergic airways disease. Proceedings of the National Academy of Sciences of the United States of America. 2009;**106**:18704-18709

[31] Kumar M, Mabalirajan U, Agrawal A, Ghosh B. Proinflammatory role of let-7 miRNAs in experimental asthma? The Journal of Biological Chemistry. 2010;**285**(le19) author reply le20

[32] Polikepahad S, Knight JM, Naghavi AO, Oplt T, Creighton CJ, Shaw C, et al. Proinflammatory role for let-7 microRNAS in experimental asthma. The Journal of Biological Chemistry. 2010;**285**:30139-30149

[33] Kumar M, Ahmad T, Sharma A, Mabalirajan U, Kulshreshtha A, Agrawal A, et al. Let-7 microRNA-mediated regulation of IL-13 and allergic airway inflammation. The Journal of Allergy and Clinical Immunology. 2011;**128**:1077-1085.e1071-1010

[34] Mayoral RJ, Deho L, Rusca N, Bartonicek N, Saini HK, Enright AJ, et al. MiR-221 influences effector functions and actin cytoskeleton in mast cells. PLoS One. 2011;**6**:e26133

[35] Mayoral RJ, Pipkin ME, Pachkov M, van Nimwegen E, Rao A, Monticelli S. MicroRNA-221-222 regulate the cell cycle in mast cells. Journal of Immunology. 2009;**182**:433-445

[36] Li JJ, Tay HL, Maltby S, Xiang Y, Eyers F, Hatchwell L, et al. MicroRNA-9 regulates steroid-resistant airway hyperresponsiveness by reducing protein phosphatase 2A activity. The Journal of Allergy and Clinical Immunology. 2015;**136**:462-473

[37] Di Valentin E, Crahay C, Garbacki N, Hennuy B, Gueders M, Noel A, et al. New asthma biomarkers: Lessons from murine models of acute and chronic asthma. American Journal of Physiology. Lung Cellular and Molecular Physiology. 2009;**296**:L185-L197

[38] Haj-Salem I, Fakhfakh R, Berube JC, Jacques E, Plante S, Simard MJ, et al. MicroRNA-19a enhances proliferation of bronchial epithelial cells by targeting TGFbetaR2 gene in severe asthma. Allergy. 2015;**70**:212-219

[39] Liao G, Panettieri RA, Tang DD. MicroRNA-203 negatively regulates c-Abl, ERK1/2 phosphorylation, and proliferation in smooth muscle cells. Physiological Reports. 2015;**3**

[40] Chiba Y, Tanabe M, Goto K, Sakai H, Misawa M. Down-regulation of miR-133a contributes to up-regulation of Rhoa in bronchial smooth muscle cells. American Journal of Respiratory and Critical Care Medicine. 2009;**180**:713-719

[41] Yamamoto M, Singh A, Ruan J, Gauvreau GM, O'Byrne PM, Carlsten CR, et al. Decreased miR-192 expression in peripheral blood of asthmatic individuals undergoing an allergen inhalation challenge. BMC Genomics. 2012;**13**:655

[42] Gaffen SL, Jain R, Garg AV, Cua DJ. The IL-23-IL-17 immune axis: From mechanisms to therapeutic testing. Nature Reviews Immunology. 2014;**14**:585-600

[43] Korn T, Bettelli E, Oukka M, Kuchroo VK. IL-17 and Th17 cells. Annual Review of Immunology. 2009;**27**:485-517

[44] Weaver CT, Elson CO, Fouser LA, Kolls JK. The Th17 pathway and

inflammatory diseases of the intestines, lungs, and skin. Annual Review of Pathology. 2013;**8**:477-512

[45] Pappu R, Rutz S, Ouyang W. Regulation of epithelial immunity by IL-17 family cytokines. Trends in Immunology. 2012;**33**:343-349

[46] Kuo G, Wu CY, Yang HY. MiR-17-92 cluster and immunity. Journal of the Formosan Medical Association. 2019;**118**:2-6

[47] Baumjohann D, Kageyama R, Clingan JM, Morar MM, Patel S, de Kouchkovsky D, et al. The microRNA cluster miR-17 approximately 92 promotes TFH cell differentiation and represses subset-inappropriate gene expression. Nature Immunology. 2013;**14**:840-848

[48] Honardoost MA, Naghavian R, Ahmadinejad F, Hosseini A, Ghaedi K. Integrative computational mRNA-miRNA interaction analyses of the autoimmune-deregulated miRNAs and well-known Th17 differentiation regulators: An attempt to discover new potential miRNAs involved in Th17 differentiation. Gene. 2015;**572**:153-162

[49] Kastle M, Bartel S, Geillinger-Kastle K, Irmler M, Beckers J, Ryffel B, et al. microRNA cluster 106a~363 is involved in T helper 17 cell differentiation. Immunology. 2017;**152**:402-413

[50] Montoya MM, Maul J, Singh PB, Pua HH, Dahlstrom F, Wu N, et al. A distinct inhibitory function for miR-18a in Th17 cell differentiation. Journal of Immunology. 2017;**199**:559-569

[51] Daniel E, Roff A, Hsu MH, Panganiban R, Lambert K, Ishmael F. Effects of allergic stimulation and glucocorticoids on miR-155 in CD4(+) T-cells. American Journal of Clinical and Experimental Immunology. 2018;7:57-66

[52] van den Berge M, Tasena H. Role of microRNAs and exosomes in asthma. Current Opinion in Pulmonary Medicine. 2019;**25**:87-93

[53] Li F, Huang Y, Huang YY, Kuang YS, Wei YJ, Xiang L, et al. MicroRNA-146a promotes IgE class switch in B cells via upregulating 14-3-3sigma expression. Molecular Immunology. 2017;**92**:180-189

[54] Chen L, Xu J, Chu X, Ju C. MicroRNA-98 interferes with thrombospondin 1 expression in peripheral B cells of patients with asthma. Bioscience Reports. 2017;**37**

[55] Recaldin T, Hobson PS, Mann EH, Ramadani F, Cousins DJ, Lavender P, et al. miR-29b directly targets activation-induced cytidine deaminase in human B cells and can limit its inappropriate expression in naive B cells. Molecular Immunology. 2018;**101**:419-428

[56] Xu H, Gu LN, Yang QY, Zhao DY, Liu F. MiR-221 promotes IgE-mediated activation of mast cells degranulation by PI3K/Akt/PLCgamma/Ca^{2+} pathway. Journal of Bioenergetics and Biomembranes. 2016;**48**:293-299

[57] Wang Q, Zhao DY, Xu H, Zhou H, Yang QY, Liu F, et al. Down-regulation of microRNA-223 promotes degranulation via the PI3K/Akt pathway by targeting IGF-1R in mast cells. PLoS One. 2015;**10**:e0123575

[58] Niu R, Xiao X, Liu B, Li Y, Zhong Y, Ma L. Inhibition of airway inflammation in a cockroach allergen model of asthma by agonists of miRNA-33b. Scientific Reports. 2017;**7**:7409

[59] Molnar V, Ersek B, Wiener Z, Tombol Z, Szabo PM, Igaz P, et al. MicroRNA-132 targets HB-EGF upon IgE-mediated activation in murine and human mast cells. Cellular and Molecular Life Sciences. 2012;**69**:793-808

[60] Qayum AA, Paranjape A, Abebayehu D, Kolawole EM, Haque TT, McLeod JJ, et al. IL-10-induced miR-155 targets SOCS1 to enhance IgE-mediated mast cell function. Journal of Immunology. 2016;**196**:4457-4467

[61] Zhou Y, Yang Q, Xu H, Zhang J, Deng H, Gao H, et al. miRNA-221-3p enhances the secretion of interleukin-4 in mast cells through the phosphatase and tensin homolog/p38/nuclear factor-kappaB pathway. PLoS One. 2016;**11**:e0148821

[62] Yang Q, Xu H, Yang J, Zhou Y, Zhao D, Liu F. MicroRNA-223 affects IL-6 secretion in mast cells via the IGF1R/PI3K signaling pathway. International Journal of Molecular Medicine. 2016;**38**:507-512

[63] Yamazumi Y, Sasaki O, Imamura M, Oda T, Ohno Y, Shiozaki-Sato Y, et al. The RNA binding protein Mex-3B is required for IL-33 induction in the development of allergic airway inflammation. Cell Reports. 2016;**16**:2456-2471

[64] Zheng J, Jiang HY, Li J, Tang HC, Zhang XM, Wang XR, et al. MicroRNA-23b promotes tolerogenic properties of dendritic cells in vitro through inhibiting Notch1/NF-kappaB signalling pathways. Allergy. 2012;**67**:362-370

[65] Maes T, Cobos FA, Schleich F, Sorbello V, Henket M, De Preter K, et al. Asthma inflammatory phenotypes show differential microRNA expression in sputum. The Journal of Allergy and Clinical Immunology. 2016;**137**:1433-1446

[66] Trinh HKT, Pham DL, Kim SC, Kim RY, Park HS, Kim SH. Association of the miR-196a2, miR-146a, and miR-499 polymorphisms with asthma phenotypes in a Korean population. Molecular Diagnosis & Therapy. 2017;**21**:547-554

[67] Hammad Mahmoud Hammad R, Hamed D, Eldosoky M, Ahmad A, Osman HM, Abd Elgalil HM, et al. Plasma microRNA-21, microRNA-146a and IL-13 expression in asthmatic children. Innate Immunity. 2018;**24**:171-179

[68] Rodrigo-Munoz JM, Canas JA, Sastre B, Rego N, Greif G, Rial M, et al. Asthma diagnosis using integrated analysis of eosinophil microRNAs. Allergy. Mar 2018;**74**(3):507-517

[69] Shapouri-Moghaddam A, Mohammadian S, Vazini H, Taghadosi M, Esmaeili SA, Mardani F, et al. Macrophage plasticity, polarization, and function in health and disease. Journal of Cellular Physiology. 2018;**233**:6425-6440

[70] Karo-Atar D, Itan M, Pasmanik-Chor M, Munitz A. MicroRNA profiling reveals opposing expression patterns for miR-511 in alternatively and classically activated macrophages. The Journal of Asthma. 2015;**52**:545-553

[71] Porta C, Riboldi E, Ippolito A, Sica A. Molecular and epigenetic basis of macrophage polarized activation. Seminars in Immunology. 2015;**27**:237-248

[72] Weiss G, Schaible UE. Macrophage defense mechanisms against intracellular bacteria. Immunological Reviews. 2015;**264**:182-203

[73] Singh SP, Chand HS, Langley RJ, Mishra N, Barrett T, Rudolph K, et al. Gestational exposure to sidestream (secondhand) cigarette smoke promotes transgenerational epigenetic transmission of exacerbated allergic asthma and bronchopulmonary dysplasia. Journal of Immunology. 2017;**198**:3815-3822

[74] Croston TL, Lemons AR, Beezhold DH, Green BJ. MicroRNA regulation of

host immune responses following fungal exposure. Frontiers in Immunology. 2018;**9**:170

[75] Xiang Y, Eyers F, Herbert C, Tay HL, Foster PS, Yang M. MicroRNA-487b is a negative regulator of macrophage activation by targeting IL-33 production. Journal of Immunology. 2016;**196**:3421-3428

[76] Montagner S, Orlandi EM, Merante S, Monticelli S. The role of miRNAs in mast cells and other innate immune cells. Immunological Reviews. 2013;**253**:12-24

Chapter 9

Nutritional Recommendations in Asthmatic Patients

Marzie Zilaee and Seyed Ahmad Hosseini

Abstract

Asthma is a heterogeneous disease, and airway inflammation has an important role in its pathogenesis. Some nutritional factors can influence the process of asthma. It is reported that saffron has anti-inflammatory, antioxidant, and muscle relaxant effects, and some animal and human studies showed that saffron and its active components (safranal and crocin) improved the asthma biomarkers and clinical symptoms. Some other nutritional factors also affect asthma; for example, magnesium can relax the muscles and thus has bronchodilatory effects. Curcumin is the major active component of turmeric which has a potent antioxidant, anti-inflammatory, and anti-allergic effects. Because some researchers suggested that intestinal microbial flora has an important role in allergy, probiotics can be a complementary supplement for asthmatic patients. Generally nutritional factors could be advised for asthmatic patients with the goal of reducing the needs for chemical drugs.

Keywords: asthma, inflammation, spirometry, nutritional recommendations

1. Introduction

Asthma is usually associated with chronic inflammation of airway [1]. In asthmatic patients, bronchial hyper-responsiveness, airway inflammation, and also airway remodeling are the prominent features. This chronic respiratory disease affects over 300 million people worldwide, and it is estimated that it will probably become more than 400 million by 2020 [2]. The WHO has estimated that 15 million disability-adjusted life-years are lost annually due to asthma [3]. Asthma disease imposes many economic and social burdens [4].

Nutritional advices have an important role in the improvement of lung function of asthmatic patients.

2. Saffron and asthma

Saffron (*Crocus sativus* L.) has antioxidant [5], anti-inflammatory [6], and muscle relaxant effects [7] and so has beneficial effects on asthma. Results of our clinical trial showed that saffron supplementation (100 mg of dried saffron stigma in capsules) for 8 weeks in mild and moderate allergic asthmatic patients improved the lung function by increasing the forced expiratory volume in 1 second (FEV_1), forced vital capacity (FVC), FEV_1/FVC ratio, and forced expiratory flow (FEF) 25-75 and decreased some inflammatory factors (anti-HSP 70 and hs-CRP) in comparison to placebo [8]. In this trial the clinical symptoms of patients (including frequency of the shortness of breath during day- and nighttime, use of salbutamol spray, waking up due to asthma symptoms, and activity limitation) improved after saffron supplementation [9].

Some animal studies also investigated the effects of saffron on asthma. Active constituents of saffron (safranal and crocin) have antioxidant and anti-inflammatory effects and so have beneficial effects on asthma. This is reported that saffron supplementation in animals with allergic asthma decreased eosinophils, basophils, and total white blood cells, and some of these effects were found to be equal to dexamethasone [10]. Saffron supplementation in guinea pig with allergic asthma decreased the serum level of endothelin1 (as an inflammatory index) [11]. Boskabady et al. reported that saffron had a potent relaxant effect on tracheal chains of guinea pigs which was comparable to or even higher than that of theophylline [7].

3. Magnesium and asthma

Insufficient magnesium (Mg) intake can influence the management of asthma [12, 13]. Some drugs used in the treatment of asthma reduce the body's magnesium storage [14]. For example, β2-receptor agonist drugs can increase urinary excretion of magnesium and thus lead to magnesium deficiency [15].

Magnesium has muscle relaxant effects and bronchodilator effects [16] because of physiologic calcium antagonist effects [17] or adenylyl cyclase activation action [18]. Results of a clinical trial on 112 patients with mild to moderate asthma suggested that 340 mg $MgSO_4$ supplementation for 2 months had bronchodilation effects and improved the lung function and so can be used as an emergency treatment for asthma attack [19].

Alexandra et al. [20] surveyed the effect of magnesium in patients with mild to moderate asthma. They showed that 340 mg Mg supplementation for 6.5 months significantly increased the concentration of methacholine required to cause 20% drop in the forced expiratory volume in 1 minute (FEV1) and improved the peak expiratory flow rate (PEFR). Mg also improved the quality of life and asthma control in comparison to control group [20].

For children with moderate-to-severe asthma, magnesium seems to be beneficial. It is a safe drug to prescribe but has minor side effects reported, for example, pain and numbness at the infusion site, hypotension, epigastric or facial warmth, flushing, dry mouth, and malaise. Due to the anti-inflammatory and bronchodilating effects, magnesium can be considered as an adjuvant therapy in pediatric patients who do not respond to conventional treatment in severe manifestations of asthma. Future studies should investigate the best route of administration and the optimal dosage for most benefits [21].

Because of the difficulties in measurement and also interpretation of extracellular vs. intracellular forms of magnesium, the relationship between asthma and magnesium deficiency is unclear [15]. Some studies reported that low dietary magnesium intake (which is the major determinant in homeostasis of magnesium) may be involved in the etiology of chronic obstructive airway disease and asthma [15]. Britton et al. reported that 100 mg/d higher dietary magnesium intake was independently associated with higher FEV1 and lower bronchial hyperreactivity [22].

4. Curcumin and asthma

Curcumin is the yellow pigment of turmeric (*Curcuma longa*) (a spice) which has anti-inflammatory [23] and anti-allergic [24] and antiasthmatic [24] effects.

In a murine model of chronic asthma, it is reported that curcumin similar to dexamethasone improved histological changes of chronic asthma [23]. Subhashini et al. reported that curcumin via intranasal rout in asthmatic mice suppressed airway inflammation [24]. So, curcumin as a complementary drug in the nasal drop form (without systemic side effects) for local use can be produced.

Chauhan et al. [25] reported that in murines with chronic asthma, curcumin (without any side effects) reduced airway inflammation and remodeling. It decreased IgE, TNF-α, and Th2 responses and increased Th1 route (as a protective response) [25].

In a clinical trial, curcumin supplementation (1000 mg twice a day) in atopic asthmatic patients has no significant effect on FEV1, serum immunoglobulin E, dose of bronchodilator consumption, and asthma control in comparison to placebo [26].

Some anti-inflammatory mechanisms of curcumin include regulation of nuclear factor kB (NF-kB) (as a transcription factor), cytokines (TNF-α and IL-6), and adenosine molecules (ICAM-1) [27].

5. Macro- and micronutrients and other nutritional factors and asthma

Oxidative stress has an important role in the progress of asthma. There are some potent evidences that the oxidant-to-antioxidant ratio reduces in asthmatic patients. Oxygen and nitrogen active species have primary effect on the airway inflammation and are indicators of asthma severity [28]. So, supplementation of antioxidants in asthma has some beneficial effects on the progression and severity of disease. It seems that a diet rich in monounsaturated fats and antioxidants that counteract the oxidative stress has a protective effect in children with asthma [29].

It is suggested that antioxidant supplementation can modulate the effects of airway injury in asthmatic patients who are exposed to air pollutants such as ozone. A clinical trial in Mexico City showed that supplementation of vitamins C and E in children with moderate-to-severe asthma reduced the loss of airway function [30].

Studies have also associated selenium deficiency with asthma [31]. A reverse relationship was seen between wheezing symptoms and insufficient vitamin E intake, but the association between asthma and vitamin E was not seen. Thus more studies must be done to understand the mechanism of vitamin E in the oxidation and inflammation of asthmatic patients [32, 33]. Nuts contain selenium and vitamin E and thus are a good choice for asthmatic patients [34].

It is reported that there is an association between asthma and low serum levels of carotenoids. Supplementation of omega-3 polyunsaturated fatty acids of fish oil in asthmatic children decreased the wheezing, but into later childhood this beneficial effect did not continue. It is reported that supplementation of zinc and vitamin C also improves the lung function and asthma symptoms [29].

Conflicting results on the benefits of vitamin D supplementation have been reported. In one study low serum levels (less than 30 ng/dL) of vitamin D were related to an increase in exacerbation of asthma [35]. In another study, high doses of vitamin D supplementation were not associated with any protective effect [36].

Children with a higher than desirable body mass index (BMI) have a significant increase in the risk of development of asthma. In obese children with asthma, weight loss diets showed improvements in the lung function, control of asthma, and quality of life [37]. The effectiveness of inhaled corticosteroid drugs is low in overweight and obese asthmatic patients [38].

The nutritionists should train the overweight and obese patients about the role of weight management in asthma control, discuss about suitable energy intake and activity, and review the known food allergies. Also the nutritionist should provide high-quality protein, vitamins, and minerals in the form of small meals to reduce the risk of infection [34].

Exposure to food allergens, especially an immunoglobulin E-mediated reaction to a food protein, can cause bronchoconstriction. Complete removal of the allergenic food protein is the only dietary advice which is currently available for food allergies. Some sulfites, such as sodium and potassium sulfides (in processed foods), have been found to be a trigger for patients with asthma [39]. Some common food allergens for children include eggs, milk, seafood, peanuts, tree nuts, fish, soy, or wheat and for adults include peanuts, tree nuts, shellfish, and fish [34].

Percentage of energy intake from fat in asthmatic patients must be high, because the respiratory quotient (RQ) of fats is lower than carbohydrate and protein [33].

Prostanoid production may be affected by dietary fat composition. Observational studies (from the 1960s and 1970s) reported that in population whose diets were rich in fish oil, the incidence of asthma was low [40]. Some studies demonstrated the fish oil anti-inflammatory effects (reduced leukocyte chemotaxis and leukotriene production) in asthmatic patients [41], but results of a systematic review showed that there is no consistent effect of fish oil on lung function, asthma medication use, bronchial hyperreactivity, and asthma symptoms [40]. A review covering 26 studies (randomized, placebo-controlled, and others) reported that the effect of w-3 fatty acid supplements could not be conclusive [42].

When the immune system of infants is immature, breastfeeding protects the immunological system and in early childhood provides a modest protective effect from wheeze [43, 44]. If the duration of breastfeeding could be longer, the protective effects seem to be more. Supplementation the diet of lactating women with fish oil could be related with alteration in the immune response of neonates to allergens, and insufficient intake of zinc and vitamins D and E during pregnancy is related to increased wheezing and asthma in children up to age of 5 years old [45]. Maternal intake of vitamins E and D can modify the development of the lung of neonates [45]. It is reported that insufficient serum level of vitamin D is an index for severity of asthma in childhood [46].

Theobromine in cocoa leads to increase blood flow to the brain and so reduces coughing and is a good food choice for asthmatic patients. It is better that these patients consume less sodium in their diet. In 5–20% of asthmatics patients who are sensitive to aspirin, salicylate sensitivity is common. Some vegetables and many fruits contain salicylates. Quercetin in pears, apples, onions, berries, and oranges should be encouraged in an amount of five or more servings per week [34].

6. Botanicals, herbs, and supplements

- ASHMI, a combination of three herbal extracts (*Ganoderma lucidum* (fungal), *Sophora flavescens*, and *Glycyrrhiza uralensis* (Fabaceae species)), is used in China for antiasthma intervention [47], and in oriental cultures and Vietnam, the seaweed is used [48].

- Gamma linolenic acid (GLA; borage oil) as a dietary fatty acid without any side effects can modulate the endogenous inflammatory mediators [49].

- *Ephedra* has bronchodilator effects, but it has some side effects such as significantly increasing blood pressure and heart rate, arrhythmias, and problems with blood glucose. This has been removed from the market by the Food and Drug Administration (FDA), but some forms are available.

- Licorice, stinging nettle, gingko, and anise have not shown efficacy, and side effects of these should be evaluated [34].

- *Boswellia serrata* extract has anti-inflammatory effects due to the triterpene compounds [50]. The mechanism of anti-inflammatory properties of boswellic acids is inhibition of proteases (cathepsin G), lipoxygenases (enzyme which is responsible for the synthesis of leukotrienes), and NF-kB [51].

7. Probiotics and asthma

It is reported that the intestinal flora can affect the mucosal immunity and so may be an effective factor for allergic disease [52]. Exposure to microbial flora in early childhood can lead to a change in the Th1/Th2 ratio toward the Th1 response.

Some studies suggested that the content of intestinal flora can be different in patients with allergic disease and also in individuals who live in industrialized countries (where the prevalence of allergic disease is higher) [53–55]; patients with allergic disease have less Bifidobacteria and Lactobacilli and more Clostridia and Staphylococcus aureu [56, 57].

The World Allergy Organization in 2015 recommended the use of probiotics for prevention of allergy in:

a. Pregnant women who have children with high risk of allergy

b. Mothers lactating infants with high risk of developing allergy

c. Infants who have risk of progressing allergies [58]

Results of a meta-analysis demonstrated that there is no evidence for protective effect of perinatal probiotic administration and childhood wheeze or asthma. So there is insufficient evidence for supplementation of probiotics for the prevention of allergic disorders and asthma, and more studies are required to explore the potential relationship between probiotic and asthma [59].

Generally, probiotic consumption for prevention of asthma and allergy is based on the little evidences, and more studies are needed for exact evaluation of the role of microflora in allergic disease and for determination of the best type of probiotic for supplementation in allergic disease [60].

Author details

Marzie Zilaee[1,2] and Seyed Ahmad Hosseini[1,2]*

1 Nutrition and Metabolic Diseases Research Center, Ahvaz Jundishapur University of Medical Sciences, Ahvaz, Iran

2 Nutrition Department, Faculty of Paramedicine, Ahvaz Jundishapur University of Medical Sciences, Ahvaz, Iran

*Address all correspondence to: seyedahmadhosseini@yahoo.com

References

[1] Bateman ED, Hurd S, Barnes P, Bousquet J, Drazen J, FitzGerald M, et al. Global strategy for asthma management and prevention: GINA executive summary. The European Respiratory Journal. 2008;**31**(1):143-178

[2] Pelaia G, Vatrella A, Busceti MT, Gallelli L, Calabrese C, Terracciano R, et al. Cellular mechanisms underlying eosinophilic and neutrophilic airway inflammation in asthma. Mediators of Inflammation. 2015;**2015**:1-8

[3] Pachter LM, Weller SC, Baer RD, Garcia de Alba Garcia JE, Trotter RT, Glazer M, et al. Variation in asthma beliefs and practices among mainland Puerto Ricans, Mexican-Americans, Mexicans, and Guatemalans. The Journal of Asthma. 2002;**39**(2):119-134

[4] Rabe KF, Adachi M, Lai CK, Soriano JB, Vermeire PA, Weiss KB, et al. Worldwide severity and control of asthma in children and adults: the global asthma insights and reality surveys. The Journal of Allergy and Clinical Immunology. 2004;**114**(1):40-47

[5] Escribano J, Alonso G-L, Coca-Prados M, Fernández J-A. Crocin, safranal and picrocrocin from saffron (*Crocus sativus* L.) inhibit the growth of human cancer cells in vitro. Cancer Letters. 1996;**100**(1-2):23-30

[6] Boskabady M, Tabatabaee A, Byrami G. The effect of the extract of *Crocus sativus* and its constituent safranal, on lung pathology and lung inflammation of ovalbumin sensitized guinea-pigs. Phytomedicine. 2012;**19**(10):904-911

[7] Boskabady MA, Aslani M. Relaxant effect of *Crocus sativus* (saffron) on guinea-pig tracheal chains and its possible mechanisms. The Journal of Pharmacy and Pharmacology. 2006;**58**(10):1385-1390

[8] Hosseini SA, Zilaee M, Shoushtari MH. An evaluation of the effect of saffron supplementation on the antibody titer to heat-shock protein (HSP) 70, hsCRP and spirometry test in patients with mild and moderate persistent allergic asthma: A triple-blind, randomized placebo-controlled trial. Respiratory Medicine. 2018;**145**:28-34

[9] Zilaee M, Hosseini SA, Jafarirad S, Abolnezhadian F, Cheraghian B, Namjoyan F, et al. An evaluation of the effects of saffron supplementation on the asthma clinical symptoms and asthma severity in patients with mild and moderate persistent allergic asthma: a double-blind, randomized placebo-controlled trial. Respiratory Research. 2019;**20**(1):39

[10] Boskabady MH, Farkhondeh T. Antiinflammatory, antioxidant, and immunomodulatory effects of *Crocus sativus* L. and its main constituents. Phytotherapy Research. 2016;**30**(7):1072-1094

[11] Gholamnezhad Z, Koushyar H, Byrami G, Boskabady MH. The extract of *Crocus sativus* and its constituent safranal, affect serum levels of endothelin and total protein in sensitized guinea pigs. Iranian Journal of Basic Medical Sciences. 2013;**16**(9):1022

[12] Fogarty A, Lewis S, Scrivener S, Antoniak M, Pacey S, Pringle M, et al. Oral magnesium and vitamin C supplements in asthma: A parallel group randomized placebo-controlled trial. Clinical and Experimental Allergy. 2003;**33**(10):1355-1359

[13] Fawcett W, Haxby E, Male D. Magnesium: Physiology and pharmacology. British Journal of Anaesthesia. 1999;**83**(2):302-320

[14] Alamoudi OS. Electrolyte disturbances in patients with chronic,

stable asthma: effect of therapy. Chest. 2001;**120**(2):431-436

[15] Dacey MJ. Hypomagnesemic disorders. Critical Care Clinics. 2001;**17**(1):155-173

[16] Gourgoulianis K, Chatziparasidis G, Chatziefthimiou A, Molyvdas P-A. Magnesium as a relaxing factor of airway smooth muscles. Journal of Aerosol Medicine. 2001;**14**(3):301-307

[17] Iseri LT, French JH. Magnesium: Nature's physiologic calcium blocker. American Heart Journal. 1984;**108**(1):188-193

[18] Brandt D, Ross E. Catecholamine-stimulated GTPase cycle. Multiple sites of regulation by beta-adrenergic receptor and Mg^{2+} studied in reconstituted receptor-Gs vesicles. The Journal of Biological Chemistry. 1986;**261**(4):1656-1664

[19] Hosseini SA, Fathi N, Tavakkol H, Yadollahpour A. Investigating the effects of oral magnesium citrate supplement on lung function, magnesium level and interlukine-17 in patients with asthma. International Journal of Pharmaceutical Research and Allied Sciences. 2016;**5**(2):86-92

[20] Kazaks AG, Uriu-Adams JY, Albertson TE, Shenoy SF, Stern JS. Effect of oral magnesium supplementation on measures of airway resistance and subjective assessment of asthma control and quality of life in men and women with mild to moderate asthma: A randomized placebo controlled trial. The Journal of Asthma. 2010;**47**(1):83-92

[21] Bichara MD, Goldman RD. Magnesium for treatment of asthma in children. Canadian Family Physician. 2009;**55**(9):887-889

[22] Britton J, Pavord I, Richards K, Wisniewski A, Knox A, Lewis S, et al. Dietary magnesium, lung function, wheezing, and airway hyper-reactivity in a random adult population sample. The Lancet. 1994;**344**(8919):357-362

[23] Karaman M, Firinci F, Cilaker S, Uysal P, Tugyan K, Yilmaz O, et al. Anti-inflammatory effects of curcumin in a murine model of chronic asthma. Allergologia et Immunopathologia. 2012;**40**(4):210-214

[24] Chauhan PS, Kumari S, Kumar JP, Chawla R, Dash D, Singh M, et al. Intranasal curcumin and its evaluation in murine model of asthma. International Immunopharmacology. 2013;**17**(3):733-743

[25] Chauhan PS, Dash D, Singh R. Intranasal curcumin attenuates airway remodeling in murine model of chronic asthma. International Immunopharmacology. 2014;**21**(1):63-75

[26] Kim DH, Phillips JF, Lockey RF. Oral curcumin supplementation in patients with atopic asthma. Allergy & Rhinology. 2011;**2**(2):e51-e53

[27] Lelli D, Sahebkar A, Johnston TP, Pedone C. Curcumin use in pulmonary diseases: State of the art and future perspectives. Pharmacological Research. 2017;**115**:133-148

[28] Sahiner UM, Birben E, Erzurum S, Sackesen C, Kalayci O. Oxidative stress in asthma. World Allergy Organization Journal. 2011;**4**(10):151

[29] Garcia-Marcos L, Castro-Rodriguez J, Weinmayr G, Panagiotakos D, Priftis K, Nagel G. Influence of Mediterranean diet on asthma in children: A systematic review and meta-analysis. Pediatric Allergy and Immunology. 2013;**24**(4):330-338

[30] Romieu I, Sienra-Monge JJ, Ramírez-Aguilar M, Téllez-Rojo MM, Moreno-Macías H, Reyes-Ruiz NI,

et al. Antioxidant supplementation and lung functions among children with asthma exposed to high levels of air pollutants. American Journal of Respiratory and Critical Care Medicine. 2002;**166**(5):703-709

[31] Allan K, Devereux G. Diet and asthma: nutrition implications from prevention to treatment. Journal of the American Dietetic Association. 2011;**111**(2):258-268

[32] Fabian E, Pölöskey P, Kósa L, Elmadfa I, Réthy LA. Nutritional supplements and plasma antioxidants in childhood asthma. Wiener Klinische Wochenschrift. 2013;**125**(11-12):309-315

[33] Mahan LK, Raymond JL. Krause's Food & The Nutrition Care Process. Elsevier Health Sciences; 2016

[34] Escott-Stump S. Nutrition and Diagnosis-Related Care. Lippincott Williams & Wilkins; 2008

[35] Brehm JM, Schuemann B, Fuhlbrigge AL, Hollis BW, Strunk RC, Zeiger RS, et al. Serum vitamin D levels and severe asthma exacerbations in the Childhood Asthma Management Program study. The Journal of Allergy and Clinical Immunology. 2010;**126**(1):52-58

[36] Litonjua AA, Lange NE, Carey VJ, Brown S, Laranjo N, Harshfield BJ, et al. The Vitamin D Antenatal Asthma Reduction Trial (VDAART): Rationale, design, and methods of a randomized, controlled trial of vitamin D supplementation in pregnancy for the primary prevention of asthma and allergies in children. Contemporary Clinical Trials. 2014;**38**(1):37-50

[37] Jensen M, Gibson P, Collins C, Hilton J, Wood L. Diet-induced weight loss in obese children with asthma: A randomized controlled trial. Clinical and Experimental Allergy. 2013;**43**(7):775-784

[38] Sutherland ER, Lehman EB, Teodorescu M, Wechsler ME, Heart N. Body mass index and phenotype in subjects with mild-to-moderate persistent asthma. The Journal of Allergy and Clinical Immunology. 2009;**123**(6):1328-1334

[39] Gaur P. Nutritional scenario in bronchial asthma. International Journal of Current Microbiology and Applied Sciences. 2013;**2**:119

[40] Shils ME, Shike M. Modern Nutrition in Health and Disease. Lippincott Williams & Wilkins; 2012

[41] Calder PC. n-3 Polyunsaturated fatty acids, inflammation, and inflammatory diseases. The American Journal of Clinical Nutrition. 2006;**83**(6):1505S-1519S

[42] Schachter HM, Reisman J, Tran K, Dales B, Kourad K, Barnes D, et al. Health effects of omega-3 fatty acids on asthma: Summary. In: AHRQ Evidence Report Summaries. US: Agency for Healthcare Research and Quality; 2004

[43] Kim J-H, Ellwood PE, Asher MI. Diet and asthma: Looking back, moving forward. Respiratory Research. 2009;**10**(1):49

[44] Oddy WH, Sherriff JL, de Klerk NH, Kendall GE, Sly PD, Beilin LJ, et al. The relation of breastfeeding and body mass index to asthma and atopy in children: A prospective cohort study to age 6 years. American Journal of Public Health. 2004;**94**(9):1531-1537

[45] Devereux G. Early life events in asthma-diet. Pediatric Pulmonology. 2007;**42**(8):663-673

[46] Brehm JM, Celedón JC, Soto-Quiros ME, Avila L, Hunninghake GM, Forno E, et al. Serum vitamin D levels and markers of severity of childhood asthma in Costa Rica. American Journal of

Respiratory and Critical Care Medicine. 2009;**179**(9):765-771

[47] Wen M-C, Wei C-H, Hu Z-Q, Srivastava K, Ko J, Xi S-T, et al. Efficacy and tolerability of antiasthma herbal medicine intervention in adult patients with moderate-severe allergic asthma. The Journal of Allergy and Clinical Immunology. 2005;**116**(3):517-524

[48] Hong DD, Hien HTM. Nutritional analysis of Vietnamese seaweeds for food and medicine. BioFactors. 2004;**22**(1-4):323-325

[49] Ziboh VA, Naguwa S, Vang K, Wineinger J, Morrissey BM, McIntyre J, et al. Suppression of leukotriene B 4 generation by ex-vivo neutrophils isolated from asthma patients on dietary supplementation with gammalinolenic acid-containing borage oil: Possible implication in asthma. Clinical and Developmental Immunology. 2004;**11**(1):13-21

[50] Ammon H. Boswellic acids in chronic inflammatory diseases. Planta Medica. 2006;**72**(12):1100-1116

[51] Ferrara T, De Vincentiis G, Di Pierro F. Functional study on Boswellia phytosome as complementary intervention in asthmatic patients. European Review for Medical and Pharmacological Sciences. 2015;**19**(19):3757-3762

[52] Ouwehand AC. Antiallergic effects of probiotics. The Journal of Nutrition. 2007;**137**(3):794S-797S

[53] Kirjavainen P, Arvola T, Salminen S, Isolauri E. Aberrant composition of gut microbiota of allergic infants: A target of bifidobacterial therapy at weaning? Gut. 2002;**51**(1):51-55

[54] Kirjavainen PV, Apostolou E, Arvola T, Salminen SJ, Gibson GR, Isolauri E. Characterizing the composition of intestinal microflora as a prospective treatment target in infant allergic disease. FEMS Immunology and Medical Microbiology. 2001;**32**(1):1-7

[55] Björkstén B. The gastrointestinal flora and the skin–Is there a link? Pediatric Allergy and Immunology. 2001;**12**:51-55

[56] Sepp E, Julge K, Mikelsaar M, Björkstén B. Intestinal microbiota and immunoglobulin E responses in 5-year-old Estonian children. Clinical and Experimental Allergy. 2005;**35**(9):1141-1146

[57] Voor T, Julge K, Böttcher M, Jenmalm M, Duchén K, Björkstén B. Atopic sensitization and atopic dermatitis in Estonian and Swedish infants. Clinical and Experimental Allergy. 2005;**35**(2):153-159

[58] Fiocchi A, Pawankar R, Cuello-Garcia C, Ahn K, Al-Hammadi S, Agarwal A, et al. World Allergy Organization-McMaster University guidelines for allergic disease prevention (GLAD-P): probiotics. World Allergy Organization Journal. 2015;**8**(1):1

[59] Azad MB, Coneys JG, Kozyrskyj AL, Field CJ, Ramsey CD, Becker AB, et al. Probiotic supplementation during pregnancy or infancy for the prevention of asthma and wheeze: Systematic review and meta-analysis. British Medical Journal. 2013;**347**:f6471

[60] Mennini M, Dahdah L, Artesani MC, Fiocchi A, Martelli A. Probiotics in asthma and allergy prevention. Frontiers in Pediatrics. 2017;**5**:165